FOR THE LOVE OF OUR CHILDREN

True Stories of Hope and Healing

By Rose-Anne Partridge

Cover Design by Gabriel Akinrinmade
Editing by Kristiana Kumpunen

Ordering Information:
For information on ordering copies of the book or bulk purchases, please contact Rose-Anne Partridge at roseanne@reallifechanges.com.

For the Love of Our Children by Rose-Anne Partridge
ISBN: 978-1-71-652585-8
First Edition

Table of Contents

Acknowledgements

When I first came up with the idea of writing this book over 10 years ago, I snatched the domain name right away. I just knew the title of this book was perfect because everything I had been doing since I became a mom was for the love of my children. I started writing immediately and then felt overwhelmed by all the information I wanted to share, and I knew I wanted to start immediately. Then, one day someone said to me, "Who would listen to your advice? You're just a mom!". Back then, I used to take these types of comments seriously, which in turn, prevented me from sharing from my heart.

I realized however, that my feelings of overwhelm and urgency were a sign to me about this book. I needed help sharing this information. Perhaps, since I was "just a mom", I needed help from experts. So I reached out to a bunch of experts in medicine, natural health, and parenting. I compiled their information, and my first "For the Love of Our Children" ebook was born. The information was great. Yet, something still didn't seem quite right, not quite enough.

That's when I had my "aha" moment. The moment I realized that I needed to reach out to a different group of experts. The ones that so many people dismiss because they don't have official titles and degrees beside their names. Moms and dads are the experts on the topic of their children. And moms and dads of children with special needs are no exception. In fact, they tend to dive deep into research and observation more so than the average person —and they are the ones going through all the challenges and observing the successful moments—so who better to ask for information than parents who have already "been there, done that"?

I am so grateful for the parents who were able to contribute to this book. They understood my vision and understood the absolute necessity for this book. Together, our voices and our journeys make a much more complete "roadmap" for others who are just starting out, or even for those who are looking to make a change of direction in their current plan of action in order to help their children live to their fullest potential. So, again, thank you to all of my fabulous and brave co-authors who jumped out of their comfort zones, staying up late or got up early to write down their stories to share. I know it wasn't easy, and yet I also know it provided you all with a wonderful outlet for your thoughts and emotions that you have been wanting to share as much as I have over the years.

I am also grateful for Michelle LeRoy with whom I have been discussing this vision for many years. When the opportunity came, she jumped on board to help me find so many of our lovely co-authors. Thank you for your words of wisdom, your optimism, your unique perspective, and your work that you have been doing for so long to help families connect on such deep levels of understanding and love with each other.

And thank you to my daughter, Kristiana, who eagerly jumped on board to help me with the editing. Having her eyes and energy as part of this project makes it even more special for me. She has always been such a help with her little brother since the day he was born. I always said that it was as if she knew right from her birth that Johan would soon be arriving, and she learned everything so fast in order to make the journey easier for me once he was here. She is a wonderfully independant, creative, and strong soul who cares for her family immensely, and we are all blessed to have her in our lives.

My wonderful husband, John, has been silently watching me work on this book for 10 years now, and I am forever grateful for the love and support he has given me and my children. He stepped into the role of stepdad with Johan with such strength and knowing. His encouragement and drive allowed Johan to truly blossom, as he is never letting Johan get away with less than what he is truly capable of accomplishing. It was interesting to see from my perspective, as Johan has always had a way of tricking me by making me believe he couldn't do as much as he could. John is the strong male role model that Johan needed in his life, and I am forever grateful that our paths lead us back to each other.

And most of all, I am so thankful that my son Johan chose me to be his mom. He has been such a guiding light for me over all these years and whenever I need a reminder for what living in joy is all about, I just need to look at him. His gentle soul has been a source of comfort and love for so many people. I am blessed to have had such an amazing teacher.

And finally, this book would not have been accomplished without our donors. I came up with the idea of a Kickstarter Campaign when working with a publisher was proving to be much too restrictive. It was a difficult decision because it put the entire project in my lap just when I thought one of my main life lessons was to learn to delegate more. However, deep down in my heart I knew it was the right choice for the overall integrity and energy of the book. And sure enough, when we reached out to have financial support through our campaign, I was brought to tears several times by all the support that came flowing our way.

Some donors have chosen to remain anonymous, but I know who they are and my heart overflows with gratitude. However, despite their request, I wanted to acknowledge their contribution in some way here in this book. So thank you, once again.

To my other donors who helped in whatever way you could, thank you! All contributions have brought this idea to becoming reality.

Kickstarter Campaign Supporters (in alphabetical order):

Arlene Anisman
Lia Bandola
Nancy Cerelli
Valerie Coates
Sabina Devita
Veronica Gaboury
Anna Grossi
Rita & Greg Haines
Danella Hesler
Susan Howson
Juha Kumpunen
Marlene Marco
Diana Mostoway
Tricia Novak
Kathy Puzic
Darcelle Runciman
Wendy Sharma
Angela Shim
Rhona Smith
Thomas Theoret
Shayne Traviss
Roy & Shirley Turunen
Risto & Laurie Turunen
Anna van Dyk

And thank you to all those who have purchased a copy of the book.

Foreword

By Michelle LeRoy

I truly was both excited and humbled by the privilege of writing the forward to this book. This book has been a decade in the making and a dream in the heart of Rose-Anne. To be able to bring to life, as well as being a platform for parents who contributed in order to share their stories, this book represents a combination of a multitude of desires to support the special needs community in a way that helps each individual to feel less isolated, to know that they are not alone in their daily struggles and stresses, and that there are countless other families out there navigating the unchartered territory of raising a child with special needs. It is a wonderful example of the vast array of similarities that are weaved throughout families dealing with special needs, while simultaneously demonstrating the uniqueness and individuality of each situation.

My name is Michelle LeRoy, a mother of three adult children, a member of Young Living Essential Oils since 2009 and an independent distributor since 2012 after witnessing all the personal triumphs and outcomes and benefits for myself and my family after the first few years of inviting these products into our lives and embracing this lifestyle. I am also a Kids Coaching Connection Youth & Families Life Coach who graduated in 2010 and opened up a private practice serving countless youth and families with quite a few of my clientele being children and families with special needs. I then went on in 2018 to become a facilitator and trainer of the Kids Coaching Connection Program as I began to see the value of each and all parents taking the course in order for them to be more deeply connected with their children in a more holistic way. I realized the benefits of how the course supported me in my parenting, and then allowed me to help others that I felt that was simply the next step, to become the first trainer under the founder of the program in Canada.

I want to applaud each and every contributor in this book for their ability to take a very private, intimate —and oftentimes hard and devastating experiences— and share them for the sake of supporting others. I know the challenge and difficulty so many parents have sharing with others and being vulnerable in front of other people.

I am thrilled that more and more people will come to understand that there is a growing number of families who are raising children with special needs, and through this book people will have the opportunity to become more and more knowledgeable, compassionate, understanding and supportive. It is my hope that readers are able to fully immerse themselves into a day in the life of these families and become more and more willing to work together to see how we can make this world a safer, brighter, happier place for these children and their families.

As a Kids Coaching Connection Coach we know that every life is created on purpose, for a purpose and the more we can look through that lense we can begin to embrace more of not only the "special needs", but also the special gifts, talents and treasures, the lessons and the blessings these children are here to bring to our world.

Thank you again to all who made this book possible including all our sponsors and donors that allowed this book to become a reality and allow these parents to have no financial barriers to their ability when getting their stories out into the world.

Created on Purpose for A Purpose
By Michelle LeRoy

What an honor it is to be asked to be part of this project and to be among some brave women and men who have shared their story about their journey through the diagnosis of one or more of their children. Hearing their stories and struggles and that of many of the clients I serve has truly created more and more motivation and passion for me to continue to support those children and families living with a diagnosis of ASD or other special needs and exceptionalities.

As a mother of three, now adult children, I can tell you that every child is truly unique and gifted in their own way. Every child has their own set of passions and things that drive them and help them to come alive and feel their value and worth in the world. I ran a home daycare for almost 11 years as a stay-at-home mom and was able to further serve a variety of children with their own unique gifts, talents, as well as needs; from diet sensitivities, to emotional and behavioral sensitivities, and children with delayed speech etc. What I was able to experience was the vast brilliance and magnificence in *every* child and the unique way they showed up and expressed themselves in the world.

I was able to witness first-hand a variety of personalities, individual talents, gifts, and the wide array of interests that each individual child gravitated toward, as well as certain areas and activities that certain children avoided. What was notable was that the way the world wanted to mould and raise a child to be inside a limited box of expectations and "norms" was not going to be something that would truly help all children thrive. And, in fact, for many it does exactly the opposite. I truly felt that each and every child in my care needed a way to express themselves in the world that voiced who they were. Many of the things society claimed were issues or that were framed in a negative way for so many of these children in my care, I actually saw them as their super powers. I saw that labelling certain aspects of a child as bad or negative instead of getting more curious about the reason these behaviours showed up the way they did would be more harmful than helpful.

My love for children, first and foremost from becoming a mother which will always be the greatest gift God could ever give to me, and then, being allowed the opportunity to be a caregiver for other children in my home and be part of their support system was also a gift I felt truly blessed to have been given.

As my children became older, I decided to branch out beyond home daycare. During a personally challenging time in my life, I wanted to gather up more tools, tips, and techniques to further strengthen myself and my knowledge in the raising and rearing of my now preteen and teenage children. This desire lead me to take a course called Kids Coaching Connection which is a five module course that was far more than I could ever imagine. This course was truly heaven-sent and the timing could not have been better. This course allowed me to dive into my own childhood and my inner child and uncover and discover aspects about me that I could fall in love with again that I had previously allowed the world to paint in a negative way. I was able to uncover so much about myself and how my earlier experiences had such a great impact on the adult I had become, and how those would either be positive or negative in terms of how I would continue to raise my children.

I was blown away at the level of healing and clarity and rediscovery I obtained about who I truly am in my essence and at my core, and I believe it made me a better mom and equipped me with countless tools to bring forth into a difficult season of my parenting life, going from a two-parent home to a single parent family. I knew that I had to do as much as I could to put that "oxygen mask" on myself first in order to truly continue to be effective and capable to parent my children now that circumstances had changed. One of the hardest things was going from primarily a stay-at-home mom who was able to have the raising of my children as my main focus, to having to split my focus a great deal going to work full-time and juggling the day-to-day household chores and tasks, homework, emotional and physical support, and being responsible to run an entire household with three kids on my own.

I share this experience with you as I know many families with special needs and challenges also experience a high divorce rate and these day-to-day struggles are truly real for them as well, on top of the extra services and outside support required for their child or children.

Taking that course truly was a life saver and gave me a renewed sense of confidence and clarity on how I wanted to go forward as a mother. Today I feel my three adult kids are thriving in the world and chasing their dreams and feel free to live life according to who they truly are and not what the world says they need to be in order to be happy or successful. I became a mom who was able to break down so many societal constraints first for myself with my own inner child, and therefore to be able to parent from that place for my children.

After taking the course, I later discovered a longing to do more and to fully proceed in becoming a fully certified ACC accredited coach within the Kids Coaching Connection organization and open my own private practice to help other parents and children live the lives they were truly born to live. So I did just that, and the clients started pouring in.

I do feel that being lead to this course was a part of God's plan for me and being able to serve children and families outside of my own, and beyond the home daycare structure was the next step in my divine path here on earth. I truly felt that there were innate skills and abilities and gifts and talents within me that God used this course to sharpen and refine, and for that I was truly grateful. It is funny how in the middle of chaos and confusion, clarity can be found and a greater version of you can be born.

To date, I have been in private practice since 2010 and continue to serve clients worldwide, many of which, interestingly enough, are families who are living with a diagnosis of ASD or other special needs with one or more of their children. Looking back, God had been preparing me for this all along with the first two children in my home daycare being one who came to me mostly non-verbal with a huge speech delay, and the other with some physical sensitivities to foods and other substances that would irritate her skin and which created rashes etc. So, through caring for these children, I was able to understand and be aware of these types of special needs from my early twenties. God seemed to send me the children in my home daycare who would unknowingly prepare me for what I continue to do today. He knew my heart and he knew that He created me *on purpose, for a purpose.*

What I aim to do today is to help all families everywhere understand that, regardless of a diagnosis or a special need or exceptionality, every child is here for a reason, every child is created *on purpose, for a purpose.* And with the uncovering of their own unique gifts, talents and treasures we can truly provide comfort to parents and caregivers and unlock the ways we are able to set that child up for a life of success. I started so passionate about this work and began seeing huge results with the families and children I worked with, that in 2018 I was accepted by the founder of the course to be the first in Canada to take her facilitator training course and now I am able to teach the 5 module course to parents, caregivers, teachers, home daycare providers, social workers, counsellors, and countless others who work in any type of profession that deals with children. I also know that this course is for everyone who ever was a child and the impact it can have on everyone who participates in it.

For me, I was created to hear beyond words, to see deeply beyond the veil of someone's fears and masks, and to truly hear their heart and to communicate with their soul. As a child, the ability to communicate in this way seemed normal to me and I believed everyone worked in this way, until over and over again I would speak other's unspoken thoughts and the person would seem confused. My questions always seemed to trigger people and I could not understand the reason. Oftentimes I would feel misunderstood and it would lead to frustration. It was not until in my early to mid 30's I truly began to understand that the way I was wired to communicate and listen was not common. This slowly seemed to be a burden and stressor in my life to be able to hear and feel so deeply, often even incredibly painful at times. However, as I began to understand myself more and was able to manage and discern more around other people, I began to navigate this burden, which I now understand is a gift, in a way that God intended for me. I was able to use this gift in a way that helped people listen and feel more deeply within themselves first and foremost, and then also listen and feel with their interactions with others. This is what the Kids Coaching Program teaches as well. From there, I realized there were many more children like me and I was determined to find a way to help them embrace and acknowledge this unique gift and channel it in a way that would serve them best.

I also support parents through the program to be able to parent these differently-abled and gifted children to be able to create an environment of greater ease and joy for them to allow them to thrive in the world. In my work I found non-verbal children to be some of the children that have these deeper listening skills and communicate on a heart and soul level and not simply on the level of their mind.

I truly believed I was designed to work with the countless children coming into this world who are different. With the increasing numbers of these special children, I felt compelled and honored to be part of this book and to let every parent know: your child is a gift. They are here for a reason, and they will be our greatest teachers moving forward in this world. Many will be born to speak beyond words and even without words, and emanate a level of joy and unconditional love beyond their diagnosis or being differently-abled.

I truly champion bringing greater awareness and more affordable and accessible services to these families and children, and will continue to advocate for this every chance I get! We are ushering in a New World and so many of these children are leading the way, if we simply take the time to stop and listen with our hearts and souls as to the reason they are increasing in numbers.

I would like to end by saying to each and every parent out there that you are your child's superhero and child's best friend, even on the days you do not feel that way. To every parent, know that you are on the frontlines of your child's life and you will often know your child better than anyone else; so never forget that. Feel the importance of who you are and continue unlocking your God given gifts to continue to be the best advocate for your child in a world still attempting to understand the bigger picture and purpose for the increase in ASD and children being born with special needs and other exceptionalities. Know that I stand with all of you as we help to create a world where all children can not only simply survive, but *thrive.*

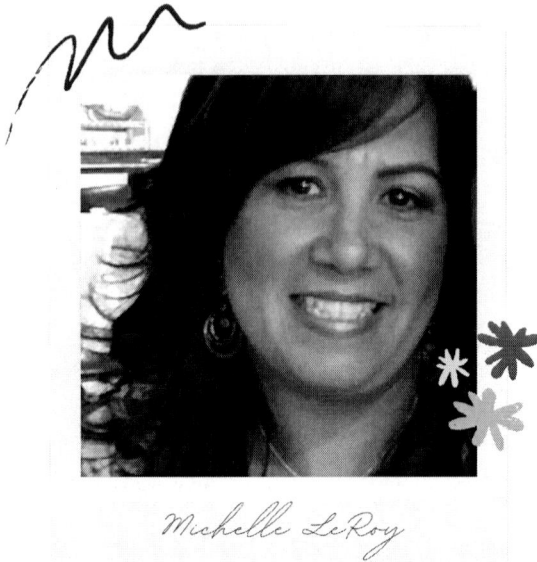

Michelle LeRoy

Michelle LeRoy is a mother of children aged 26, 24 and 20 years old. She has a passion for the health and wellbeing of children and youth, and helping parents and caregivers find pure and healthy plant based options, tools, and techniques to support their children in all areas of their lives, mentally, emotionally, physically, and spiritually. Michelle does this through her almost 10 years as an ACC Accredited Kids Coaching Connection Holistic Youth Life Coach, Facilitator, and a member of the International Coach Federation through which she has supported children, youth, and families worldwide with uncovering their own uniques gifts, talents and treasures and helping them to pursue them in the world in a way that fulfils them body, mind, and spirit. You can find her leading countless workshops and seminars along with one-on-one and group coaching whether it be families or in schools and other organizations that support the wellbeing of youth and children. Michelle has worked with children with a diagnosis of ADD, ADHD, autism, aspergers, anxiety, depression, sensory processing disorder, oppositional defiant disorder, OCD, and countless other exceptionalities and uniquenesses and is able to look beyond the diagnosis in order to establish together with the child and the child's parents and/or caregivers the most effective tips, tools, and techniques that enables a child to learn, grow and thrive in a way that honours the truth of their heart and soul. As a mindfulness meditation facilitator, Michelle holds classes for children 4 to 12, as well as teens 13 to 17 years old. She has also studied and practiced Energy Medicine which encompasses a wide array of modalities and complementary therapies in order to further support the needs of the whole child. In addition, Michelle incorporates her vast knowledge of essential oils for the well-being of children and adults alike.

Young Living Essential Oils Independent Distributor ID#1084801
Bottles Of Bliss Team
Harnessing Heaven in every drop!
www.bottlesofbliss.com
www.michelleleroy.marketingscents.com/
https://www.facebook.com/groups/BottledBlissTeam/
https://www.facebook.com/younglivingbymichelle
https://www.facebook.com/younglivingkids
https://twitter.com/YLwithmichelle

ACC Certified Kids Coaching Connection Life Coach
Member of the International Coach Federation &
Founder of The New Earth Children Centre
http://michelleleroy888.wix.com/anewearthanewchild
www.thenewearthchildrencentre.com
https://www.facebook.com/groups/newearthchildrensupport/
(416) 700-9012

SECTION ONE

Opening Comments & Disclaimer

I do not have a doctorate and cannot diagnose or prescribe anything. I am not a scientist or certified research analyst on any well-financed study. I am not a biochemist, nor an inventor developing life-changing products. And I will state it here since it will need to be said somewhere: this book is not intended to treat, cure, heal, or diagnose any disease, mental illness, or symptom. This applies to all contributions from all of its co-authors.

All that being said and clarified, what I am is, much more important in the lives of my children. I am a mother that loves her children and wants them all to have the very best of life and to reach their fullest potential, whatever that may look like in the end.

I want to share with you a little bit about this book and my intentions with it all. I have had the idea of writing this book for over 10 years. I began to write it about five years ago, however, along the way to creating this book, the original intention has changed. I was writing it all on my own, sharing our unique journey. As I was writing, I had an epiphany. This book cannot be written only by me! The book is called, *For the Love of Our Children* and the vision was to make it a roadmap for parents who have children with special needs. But, something inside me kept saying it wasn't enough yet.

The issue with many self-help style books is that they don't take into account the exceptions to the rules or the unique individuals that are our children. They don't look at the odd ones out. Most books give advice that is black and white and often linear. However, everything in real life can be messy and beautiful all at the same time. Nothing can truly prepare us for the situations that we never thought possible, or the moments no one saw coming.

Even with as much experience and knowledge that I felt I had gained over the years with my own son, Johan, I realized that our journey is unique—really unique. And yet, along our way we encountered so many other parents who have found wonderful ways to support their special children. More than a simple how-to book, *For the Love of Our Children* needed to take the perspectives of many other moms and dads on this similar path to create a better

16

and bigger roadmap to help our children to live to their fullest potential. So beyond my own story, it grew to what you see now in this book when I reached out to my community.

For my contribution to the book, I will be focusing on my wonderful journey in life as a mom. I have been compelled to study and research many alternative ways to keep my family healthy. Driven by the love I have for my children, I always do my best to find the best solutions, and I feel that because I do not have all the other official roles or titles stated in the disclaimer above, I have the ability to look at all potential solutions with an unbiased perspective due to the love and discernment that a mother innately has for her children.

One of the biggest lessons I have learned through my trials is that there is very rarely, if ever, simply *one* thing, *one* method, *one* product that is needed for my family and, in particular, for my son who has special needs. I have seen wonderful changes and progress with many different solutions. And as I write, I am still looking for more answers, more pieces to this puzzle.

I like to describe it as a puzzle: each piece of the puzzle comes together with another to make the complete picture. Without one piece of the puzzle, there is still a mystery as to what the complete picture will look like. As we get closer to placing all the pieces, this picture becomes clearer. However, in real life, even if I don't find all the pieces of the puzzle, but I find as many as I can to see the beauty of the final product, I am happy. That being said, when I know there are still more pieces scattered out there, I *will* keep looking. That's just who I am. Some pieces don't fit my son's puzzle. They will, however, fit someone else's. To me, most of the time there is no right or wrong solution in the sense of "it works" or "it doesn't work". It may simply not fit this unique puzzle that is my son's life. I have tried many things that have not worked for him that others have sworn by. Were they lying? Nope. It worked the way they needed it to, it just wasn't what he needed.

In these sections of the book I am sharing our story, our journey, and the solutions that I have found to work for my son and my family. Perhaps there is a suggestion that you have not heard about yet and it may work for your child? Maybe it won't. But, you won't know until you try. The best proof is in the results and it is my strong belief that you can only obtain results through trying.

Some may call that raising false hope. I simply call it hope. Staying true to the course and persevering through the ups and downs, all the while understanding that these so-called failures are simply part of the process and the journey. And I give thanks for each potential solution that I have tried in the past, whether it has "worked" for my son or not because it has led me to where I am now. With each trial, I am closer to finding another puzzle piece that will help him be the best he can be—healthier, stronger, and full of joy.

What this book is really about is sharing. I remember feeling alone when we first received the diagnosis, and in a way we were because it is such a rare condition. There are no support groups in my town to go to, there is even very limited information about it online. When my husband was talking about it the other day with some of his colleagues, he mentioned that when you put the official diagnosis into the search engine, my son's photo is the first image that comes up. For a long time, his photos were the only things that came up online because I was the only one writing about it and our experiences. And yet, even as rare as it is, I am definitely not alone. I am a mother of three beautiful children, one of which has special needs. I have met many wonderful mothers along the way that have similar situations, even if the labels applied to our children differ. And we share many of the emotions that follow: frustration, confusion, anger, despair, joy, and happiness along our journey with our children.

My hope is that by sharing our story, if there is another family that is going through something similar, no matter what official diagnosis they are given, they can find some comfort in knowing that there are also the good feelings that come with the situation, and that with every challenging situation that arises, there are wonderful things that can come from it all.

I am a stronger, wiser, more loving, balanced, and healthy mom because of this journey. How could I not be? All the research I have done for my son, I have applied to my life as well. To top it off, I have recently gone through being a new mom all over again. I have my 22-year-old daughter, my 21-year-old son, and now my eight-year-old boy. What a fabulous new leg of the journey that has been added to the original destination.

I believe I am a better mother to my youngest son thanks to all the knowledge I have gained over the years with my first two, and the challenges I have faced finding the best path for their health and well-being. And I know that his arrival has been a joy to my other children as well.

I feel blessed to have this story to share, and I am so thankful for all the other parents who have contributed their stories. Together, we share so much in common. While I was reading through their chapters I was moved to tears, I smiled and laughed with joy, and I took notes for things to consider for my own son. I hope this book reaches those parents who are needing it as they begin their own special journey.

The Journey of Shock and Grief Through to Joy and Hope

I had a dream. I am not talking figuratively. I actually had a dream one night. It went like this: there seemed to be a race or marathon going on with a lot of people participating. As far back as I could see and as far ahead, there were people moving along in this "race". It wasn't on a track. It didn't even stick to the roads. It seemed to meander just about anywhere, but people mostly seemed to be going on the same path. I was running along holding Johan's arm to help him along the way. Every now and then he would glance at me. Strangely though, my legs were moving really fast like I was running, however, my feet couldn't seem to find the ground. It was like I was relying on the speed of my legs to propel me through the air instead. And it was tiring. I really wanted to be able to run on the ground like everyone else.

Every now and then, one foot would feel the ground and I would push off to try to get more momentum and I would feel this rush of happiness that I actually touched. And then, once again, round and round my legs would fly like in a cartoon, trying to gain more speed.

I watched as others passed by us. My main concern was having a good hold of Johan's arm so that he wouldn't slip behind. John, my husband, was there for a moment, but he seemed to be able to touch the ground, so he was off ahead with some of his firefighting co-workers, chatting away while they raced ahead.

The path weaved in and out, over streams, through fields, and then we came to a strange new direction. There was a hollowed out tree that everyone was climbing through from the inside starting from the bottom up. I guess the tree was hanging there in mid-air somehow. When we arrived there, I knew that Johan could never climb up on his own like everyone else. It was a fairly narrow tree. Big enough for one person at a time to climb up with comfort, but it would be tight for two of us to do it together. That was the only possible way though. So, I hooked his arms around my shoulders and started to climb. It was not easy. It was tight and I struggled. He was so much bigger than he was years ago. It's no longer as easy to carry him with me. Every now and then, he would kick out his legs because it wasn't comfortable holding onto my back for so long. This made it even more challenging.

But I was doing it. Step-by-step, little by little, we moved up the tree. The strange thing was, I had no idea what was waiting above us. The farther up the tree we climbed, the darker it became. Earlier on in the race, we were always able to see what was next. I couldn't anymore. I just had to keep climbing up and holding tight so that he would not fall.

What did this dream mean? Well, I may not be a professional dream interpreter, but some ideas came to mind when I jolted awake at 4 a.m.

This race obviously represented the journey of life. And while all the others around me seemed to be moving along fine because they could "touch the ground", caring for a child who has special needs makes for more obstacles and challenges. It can be tiring, and sometimes it can feel like you are going nowhere in comparison to others, despite what seems to be a great effort in moving fast and moving forward.

The most interesting part of the dream was the tree. You see, my son is getting older now. He is 21-years-old. And even though things weren't easy when he was younger, I was still able to know, more or less, what I needed to do for him day-to-day. I could "see" the way. But now as he is in adulthood, the future is much less clear. I don't know what his future holds quite frankly. But, nonetheless, I will keep moving forward, keeping him as safe and happy as I can.

I have hope and faith that as long as I keep moving forward, there will be the next step that will be waiting for us to move us up and along our path on this journey of life.

It Started With Andrew

When I first started writing this book, I had completely forgotten about a very important phase in my life. It's a moment that makes you think that everything truly is planned out for your life. Or perhaps, it was just a very helpful coincidence. In all honesty, when I thought about it, it somewhat freaked me out—could this moment in my life have been preparing me for Johan?

Back when I was 17-years-old, my sister's friend asked me if I would be willing to take over a babysitting job that she no longer had the time to do since she was too busy in university. The pay was really good—$8 an hour. Back then, that was a lot of money for babysitting! And yes, I am dating myself with that fact. All I had to do was spend time with a little boy whose name was Andrew. The catch? He was diagnosed with autism.

What's autism? These days most people can answer that to a certain degree. Many people may also know someone with this diagnosis. The rate of autism these days is something shocking like 1 in every 150 people according to some reports. But back in 1988, it was only around 5 to 6 cases in every 10,000.

So for me to get a job taking care of someone with autism was a very rare situation. I took the job and enjoyed spending my time with Andrew. I knew all of his triggers. For example, he didn't like to change direction while walking. So if we needed to go for a walk, it would have to be around a block in order to be able to get back home. He liked to rock back and forth for comfort. Sometimes he would want to bang his head. He made loud moans when he was frustrated. He thought it was a really big treat to take the subway to go to get Chicken McNuggets. And he *loved* it when I was there to play with him.

It was such an educational experience for me. I had never met anyone like Andrew before this opportunity. I had to take a bus and subway all the way from the middle of Scarborough to the Beaches in Toronto each time I worked with him. For those not familiar with the geographical references, that is far to go for a babysitting job. He impacted my life so much that I even wrote my final Grade 12 report for physical education (en français en plus) about autism and my experiences with Andrew.

Why was this significant for me? Back then, working with children who had special needs was not as common as it is now. And strangely enough, I was thrown into that world with zero education or training on any of it. What I didn't know was that Andrew was somewhat my early training for my life with my own son.

Not a Usual Baby Story

It started early in the morning, but this time around I was much more relaxed and calm about the situation. I knew there was no point rushing to the hospital at this stage. The contractions were becoming stronger and more regular, but instead of having to pace it out in a sterile and unfamiliar setting like I did with my firstborn, I chose to pack up my one-and-a-half-year-old daughter in the stroller and walk around the neighbourhood to help things continue to progress.

By the evening, I was ready to see my doctor. I was so much calmer about this wonderful process now that it was my second time giving birth. And everything had been "textbook" with the whole pregnancy. So I knew I would be shortly holding my newborn son in my arms.

As he emerged, I could see his blonde hair and long body. All looked good from my perspective, but I caught a glance of concern on my doctor's face. He was not breathing immediately! But, that concern quickly faded as he gasped his first big breath. The nurses cleaned him up and brought him to me finally.

My beautiful boy, Johan.

Looking back, I now wonder if perhaps taking that first challenging breath was foreshadowing the challenges that would continue in my son's life. It started in the hospital shortly after his birth. For some reason, he had an underdeveloped chin. He also didn't have a rooting reflex. This made it very difficult to breastfeed, which I was determined to do better with this time around. I only managed to breastfeed my daughter for a little over three months due to limited support and insufficient information and I didn't have the resources at my fingertips like we do nowaday. Thankfully though, there were two angels in the hospital that helped me teach Johan how to latch on with tape and tubes and eventually breastfeed exclusively.

After a bout of jaundice, which I was somewhat prepared for since my daughter had it as well, we finally were released from the hospital a week after his birthday. Things were looking good and I was feeling confident that all was well.

My daughter, Kristiana, was a precocious child. She whipped through the various stages of development with lightning speed. So when it came to Johan, I didn't want to compare his development to hers. After all, we are always told that every child is unique and will develop at their own unique pace. But deep down I knew that something was not quite right. And it turned out that our family doctor agreed that he wasn't hitting his milestones in a timely manner.

So our specialist appointments began. First on the list was an ophthalmologist to better understand why Johan wasn't tracking with his eyes yet. First diagnosis: Duane syndrome. We had never heard of this syndrome but they clarified what this was for us in their official diagnosis letter:

> *Duane syndrome, also called Duane retraction syndrome (DRS), is a group of eye muscle disorders that cause abnormal eye movements. People with Duane syndrome have difficulty rotating one or both eyes outward (abduction) or inward (adduction).*

This eventually led us to his first surgeries to help correct, at minimum, his crossed eyes. It would not, however, help him to have any peripheral vision. We have also suspected over time that he has difficulty with his depth perception due to his hesitation on level changes and colour or pattern variations on the floor.

We were eventually referred to a neurologist by our paediatrician who thought it would be a good idea to take a closer look at Johan's brain through an MRI. His results provided further clues into his unique situation as they discovered issues with specific areas of his brain such as the white matter, thinning of the corpus callosum, and the myelin sheath.

The neurologist then referred us to a genetics specialist for more testing. The tests were done on my son, myself, and his biological father. We finally got a "name" for what we were dealing with: chromosome 8p inverted duplication. And with the name came a bunch of unknowns and potential extremes.

> *Johan has an inverted duplication of the short arm of chromosome 8 (the p arm). The break points are 11.2 to 23. His karyotype is written 46,XY, inv dup (8)(p11.2p23).*

Even with these new insights on his brain and this new label that was provided by the test results, we weren't given any real direction for how to help him at the time. We were as lost as we were before getting the diagnosis because there were so few cases to refer to, and each case was so unique based on how severe the individual's unique symptoms manifested.

And then, slowly over time, somehow Johan fell through the cracks of the medical institutions. Maybe it was my fault? Maybe it was due to me having "specialist burnout"? So many appointments all the time. So much waiting. However, it was suggested at the local children's centre that we may want to have Johan in a daycare setting to help him through role modeling different developmental stages for his own growth and development. Sounded like a good idea, so I placed both Kristiana and Johan into a local daycare centre.

I will always remember the day I went to introduce some of the staff to Johan and explain the challenges we had noted so far. One of the daycare providers offered to watch Johan while I went over the paperwork with the director. Hesitant, I reluctantly agreed since I was going to be letting them take care of him every weekday very soon. I quickly explained that he had just started to walk at two-and-a-half-years-old and that his balance wasn't very good, so most of the time you needed to watch him so that he doesn't fall down or get pushed over by other children. With a lack of peripheral vision, this meant he couldn't see things coming at him from the side. She reassured me that she would watch him carefully, so off I went into the office.

I was only a short moment away from him before the daycare provider came rushing into the office to get me. "He fell and hit his head!", she gasped at me. "I was watching him while he was in line with all the other children when suddenly he just went down."

Right. Just like I had explained. Sigh. This was not going to be an easy path. As much as it was challenging for us to know how to raise and help Johan, it was going to be even more so for others that were not used to having to deal with a child that needed extra mobility care, but wasn't in a wheelchair. I say that because they had mentioned that they had previously helped take care of other children with special needs that used wheelchairs as an example. Johan was mobile. Simply not steady and sturdy, especially with other more "able-bodied" children running around.

It was a solid hit to the head which happened to land right on the protruding door jam on the floor. I rushed him off to the hospital to get his first stitches to close the gaping wound that had opened up.

I was frustrated and somewhat irritated at the daycare. I know that accidents happen, but I had just explained to her that he requires extra attention. And yet, I had to somehow put this behind me and bring him back there and trust that all would be well; that this experience would benefit him and help him to continue to develop. Time to have faith.

Faith is something that I have had to dip into regularly on this journey. Faith that I would find the answers I needed for Johan. Faith that I would be able to be strong enough to keep going and be the best mother I could possibly be. Faith that I would be able to keep going against the stream of nay-sayers, pessimists, and dark prognosis, otherwise known as the "realists" who felt it was best for me to simply accept his limitations and plan and prepare for the worst.

From Baby to Boy

Daycare soon turned into school and that meant a whole new slew of tests and predictions by the professionals within that system. Don't get me wrong, whenever there was a new test or evaluation recommended or completed, deep down I was actually very grateful. For one, it made me feel that I wasn't all alone in this journey. And secondly, it gave us some new insights to work from. They weren't always helpful insights, but how would you know until you tried, right?

Take for example the psychological testing that they put him through in order to get him registered into the public school system. It showed that he was developmentally delayed–yes, we knew that. It showed that he was functioning at a level several years younger than his physical age–yes, we knew that as well. And it stated that they were unable to complete the full test due to his limitations. So, not all that helpful in the end.

The interesting thing about tests in my opinion, and this applies to everyone no matter their ability, is that test results are a product of what the individual being tested is willing to show, not just what they are capable of showing. We learned several years later that it made a big difference *how* you asked a question to Johan.

One day in Grade 4, his educational assistant was helping him to do some colouring. She asked him to colour with the red crayon. He picked up the blue one and started to colour. "Oh well," she thought, "he still doesn't know his colours. Something to work on". Continuing to colour together, she asked if he could pass her the red crayon. Johan picked up the red crayon and passed it to her. She was amazed! Was it a fluke? She continued and asked him to pass colour after colour and he got most of them correct. He knows his colours.

The only difference was the way she asked. He didn't want to colour with the red crayon. He wanted to colour with the blue one. But he was happy to help her out by passing her the crayons she needed. They continued testing this new theory with other concepts and soon discovered he knew many animals, too. The standard testing they were doing would have never shown this knowledge.

Finding My Purpose

It was probably soon after he entered school that I truly started finding my purpose. Tests and textbooks were not much help in determining the best steps forward for Johan. There was very little information on his specific condition and the more I asked questions, the more I realized I was going to have to figure out the answers myself.

So I started to research and read everything I could that was remotely related to Johan's symptoms and challenges. Through the years, there were some key areas that kept coming up as the most important to look into: the brain, the gut, his immune system, his environment, and his relationships. Book by book, course by course, I learned all that I could learn to help Johan live each day to his fullest potential; for him to shine.

Allowing Johan to Shine

When most people meet Johan and spend some time with him, they usually comment on how cheerful and easygoing he is. He is a gentle soul that loves to observe others and the world around him. He loves slapstick humour, people singing loud and off key, and he likes to play his own little pranks on people every now and then just for a giggle.

He loves animals. Horses are his favorite. I think he would love dogs and cats more (at least being around them) if he wasn't so allergic to them. He loves balls. He is actually quite good at basketball—dribbling and bouncing it away. He likes to kick and throw all sorts of balls. He loves music. I love watching his legs go into his own wacky dance steps when he likes a song playing. Joy and laughter are primary states of being for Johan.

Then, there is the young adult that he has become. He loves to sleep. He likes to watch movies—all day long if you let him. And he can trick those who don't know him well into believing he can't do as much as he can. He's not a fan of me giving away his secrets like that, but that's what moms are for. To push their children to be the best they can be, at all times. Not only when we are watching.

What I have noticed is that he really does love being in the "ethers" surrounding our physical world. Sleeping, daydreaming, zoning out. I wish I could know exactly what he does and experiences in those states. But the reality is, he lives here with us and we need him here in the physical world in order to thrive and shine in a way we can all see.

That's when I started to realize what he really needed. Johan wants to feel safe. And not just in ways that we may think of as "safe", as in security. It also means emotionally safe and environmentally safe. This means maintaining a clean environment: avoiding toxic chemicals, eating clean foods, surrounding him with love and support, but also with discipline and boundaries on top of pushing his limits, as well. It's amazing how even the fact of setting low expectations for your child with special needs can affect them emotionally, and even more amazing to notice how sensitive they are to the emotions of those around them. This one took me a while to understand: when mommy is happy, Johan is happy.

Some of Johan's greatest breakthroughs took place after I started to take care of myself, both emotionally and physically. This did mean, among many other things, getting a divorce (an all-too-common reality in families who have children with special needs it seems) and a while later, this meant welcoming a wonderful new role model for Johan when I remarried. His stepdad is truly one of the best things to happen for Johan's development. John, my husband, knows how to motivate and push Johan just enough to blow me away with his abilities. He is the one who was determined enough to get Johan to drink out of a cup, to stand up from the floor in the middle of a room on his own, to help with little chores and responsibilities. John knew he could do more than he was allowing even me to see.

I am a big advocate of parents ensuring that they are taking care of their own needs as well as their child's needs. We have all heard about caregiver burnout. But how often are we taking it to heart as we care for our child with special needs?

So as you read through the suggestions and stories in this book, I encourage you to see how you can apply some of the advice to your own health and well-being. There aren't many supplements or physical therapies that I have applied to Johan's day-to-day life that I haven't used in some way or form for myself. And I am happy to report that I am healthier, stronger, and happier now than I was at the beginning of this journey. And I have Johan to thank for the constant reminder to take care of myself first.

If this is a challenge for you to accept for your life, remember this question: who will be there to take care of your special child and your other children when they need you? Take care of yourself and your needs, and you will be there as long as they need you.

Beyond Words

Communication is more than words. It is about making meaningful exchanges and understanding intentions and emotional energy. When Johan was just a few months old I had to go to the bank and brought him along for the ride. Despite our rocky start, he was a very happy and contented baby for the most part. He liked being in the car, and he was very patient. I had him in his portable car seat sitting with me in the waiting room and he was babbling away with joy (some things never change). An older lady was also waiting there and she remarked, "Wow, he sure is a talkative baby! He is going to be quite the talker when he gets bigger."

Talking? Well, no. But communicating is the better description. Over the years, despite being nonverbal, Johan has found wonderful ways to communicate his needs and feelings through gestures, sounds, and some essential sign language.

Recently, Johan started at a new highschool because we moved. As usual, I went through all the interviews with teachers, principals, and support staff, giving all the most important information on how to work best with Johan. One of the most important topics typically is how to communicate with him. Although the list of available methods seems insufficient, after a few weeks in I always get the message sent to me that Johan sure has a way of communicating what he wants. It makes me laugh each time.

I laugh because when you do get to know him, his personality and quirks make you laugh, and the teachers always "get" what I do my best to share during the initial meetings. He grunts in disapproval with his arms crossed. He claps and laughs heartily making everyone around him smile and laugh along with him. The best joke that he loved to play daily on them was the emotions/mood check-in first thing in the morning. They have colour zones—green, yellow, and red. Green being very happy, yellow so-so, and red unhappy/angry. Without fail he always selects the red one and waits for their reaction. And when they say, "Johan, you're angry?" he laughs with joy and runs off.

Living in Joy

One of the most important things that I have personally learned with Johan is that emotions have so much energy, and that energy affects more than the individual feeling those emotions. Emotions are so important for us to understand, and supporting healthy emotions even moreso.

I already mentioned that Johan taught me that when I was happy, he was happy. This is because he is so sensitive to the energy that comes from our emotions. He may not be able to speak, but he has an uncanny ability to read people's emotions and thoughts quite telepathically. I also want to clarify that when I recommend supporting healthy emotions, I do not mean stifling or rejecting emotions such as anger, frustration, sadness, etc. It's not about being happy all the time. It's allowing your emotions to communicate to you what they need to express. Emotions are key to self-expression, and you need to listen to those emotions, process them, and then allow them to flow out and away to make room for happiness or whatever emotion serves you and your child best.

I have found that particular essential oils have the potential to assist in supporting emotional wellness. Specifically, essential oils largely affect the hypothalamus and pituitary gland, which once stimulated, release hormones into the body. So if we inhale essential oils with stimulating properties, it will produce a response in the appropriate part of the limbic system. The limbic system is a set of brain structures that plays a role in emotions, particularly those that evolved early and which play an important role in survival.

By diffusing essential oils in our home daily and topically on Johan, I have found that he is able to effectively communicate his needs without as much frustration as he has expressed in the past. Or if there is a particularly challenging day coming up for him–hospital visits, for example–using essential oils to help keep him feeling calm and relaxed helps everyone in the end. And I can assure you that I am also using all those oils to help keep me calm and strong for him at the same time.

Keep Going

I used to spend countless hours at the hospital emergency with Johan due to severe asthma reactions. I remember praying in the car during those stressful moments as I rushed him off alone, seeing his little face in the rearview mirror turning blue because he was struggling to get oxygen into his body. I knew I had to find the answers myself because the "quick fix" at the hospital would soon pass and I would be there again another day, strong on the outside but terrified on the inside. And I did figure it out. By eliminating all the harsh and toxic chemicals from our home, eliminating exposure to pets, and boosting his immune system naturally, he no longer needs his asthma medications when he is in my care.

And then repeat for the next challenge on the agenda. Scoliosis. Who knew that this would be the diagnosis to provide the biggest health hurdle for Johan? I certainly would not have guessed it with the huge list of medical issues to choose from on his unique list. We knew from around seven-years-old or so that he had a slight curvature to his spine. But it really wasn't all that noticeable. He was skinny and small in stature so it somewhat blended into his overall physique. And the doctors never really made it out to be that big of a deal. We got the necessary orthotics and supports for his legs and feet that seemed to be the bigger and more immediate physical challenges to tackle. This would suddenly and rapidly change when he turned 16.

Growth spurts began in his mid-teenage years and yet he was still so thin with low muscle tone due to his condition that we thought our biggest struggle was to find pants that were long enough for his rapidly stretching legs that could also still stay on his narrow hips. However, one day we were walking through a mall (one of his favourite places to walk due to all the visual stimulation and flat, safe surfaces for his balance) and I looked back at him smiling at all the window displays and people walking by. He had a good pace and was swinging his arms back and forth, which he does when he is happy and moving along quickly. My focus turned to my littlest who was only three at the time who was running at full speed ahead of us. Checking back to make sure Johan was keeping up I saw that suddenly he was hunched over severely and had to hold himself upright by bracing his hand on his thigh. But even with this support, he was so bent over he could barely walk. My heart sank into my gut. I turned away and started to cry, right there, in the middle of the mall, trying my best not to let Johan see my tears. John went back to help support Johan, I picked up my youngest son, and we quickly went home.

I still couldn't understand how it happened so rapidly. This obviously lead to a new slew of specialist appointments and x-rays, which Johan hated so much because the sound of the machines terrified him. We went to see a neurosurgeon at one of the best children's hospitals in the area. After examining Johan's x-rays he came in to speak with me. Johan was sitting right there beside me when he said, "There is nothing we can do. This surgery would kill him. Make him as comfortable as you can. Make sure he enjoys life. It's hard to say how much longer he will be around. As his scoliosis progresses, it will slowly crush his internal organs. Did no one prepare you for this?"

The last question was asked as he saw tears begin to stream out from my eyes uncontrollably. "No", I thought to myself, no one has ever mentioned this. Somehow, through the tears and confusion filling my mind, I managed to ask for a second opinion. A few months later, sitting in the same hospital, the second neurosurgeon confirmed that he would not be willing to risk the surgery either. This particular surgeon had a better "bedside manner" and was much kinder when he spoke to me about the situation. I was also more prepared this time and my typical mom-shield was up and functional. I was strong again and even more determined to find a solution.

And yet again we did find one. Now, I admit that I don't know how long this solution will last. But what I know is that once again I have found a way to keep my son with us and as healthy as possible at the same time. Instead of a risky surgery, we found a spinal brace to help support his body. And with this brace we went from needing a wheelchair for longer distances, to being able to walk independently almost at all times. He is mobile again which allows his legs to keep strong. We also have a walker which he can sit on for breaks for when we travel.

The funny thing about Johan is that he loved the wheelchair while he was using it. He loves the walker when we pull it out for support. And he is fine with walking around on his own. At least when he isn't having a lazy moment. And lately I have been pushing him out of his comfort zone more and more. Instead of safe, flat surfaces such as streets and sidewalks, we have been going more adventurous and taking walks through forest trails. Definitely more challenging for both of us as I need to be closer to him to help him avoid roots and rocks and uneven dips. But he loves being right in the middle of nature with us. He loves being included in our adventures. So we will keep going. We will continue to face each new challenge as they come. There may be more tears, but I will always find the next solution to move us forward. As I have already stated, there is no such thing as false hope in my mind. Have hope! It will be the key ingredient that will support your inner strength to stay the course, no matter what you are dealing with at each moment.

SECTION TWO:

Collective Voices of Hope and Inspiration

I am a firm believer in the concept of "it takes a village to raise a child". And while our society may seem to have drifted apart in many ways, I think there is a way to still tap into our collective power by sharing our wisdom and our stories. Sharing experiences through storytelling is an effective way to exchange and consolidate knowledge. Storytelling has been an ancient means of passing on wisdom. It builds trust, cultivates norms, transfers tacit knowledge, and facilitates unlearning, and emotional connections. And yes, there is a lot of information that we need to unlearn, as much as there is information to learn.

I am so grateful for the parents who agreed to share their stories to help create this "roadmap" of wisdom that we can hopefully pass on to those starting on their special journey. When I was reading through these for the first time, even at my stage of the game, it brought me to tears. The feeling of understanding and "I get that!" moments for my own life brought me such comfort and feelings of connection.

Trust in the Journey

By Susan Baker

If you had told me this was how our story would unfold, I wouldn't have believed you. Our journey began 12 years ago with the birth of our first-born child—though you might say it began 20 years ago when I first became a holistic nutritionist, or even 40+ years ago when I, myself, entered the world. It is all part of the same journey.

I'm Susan, author of the blog Life, Love & Autism, with a 20 year background in holistic health and nutrition. Mom to Andrew (12, nonspeaking, on the autism spectrum) and Abby (eight years, and very much speaking), at the time of this writing. We live in Toronto, Canada. I am not an expert on autism, but I can share what I've learned and experienced so far—maybe so that others can learn from it, too.

With our first-born, it was all new. Was it? Wasn't it? But by age two,, our son's development looked atypical. By three, we were in "early intervention services", and by four years old, he was diagnosed with autism spectrum disorder (ASD). To me, he was always my beautiful, unique Andrew.

What I didn't see was the incredible journey that lay ahead. As I said before, I wouldn't have guessed it. I expected it would look something more like this: I would continue to explore natural, holistic therapies. We'd do brain-body work. We'd go deeper into nutrition. We'd do another heavy metal cleanse, and a deep metabolic reset. I'd uncover the natural remedy, 'the missing piece', and one day, my child would emerge; one day it wouldn't look like autism.

If I'm honest, that's how I thought it would go. I know this is possible with some kids; I expected it with mine. I do know that the therapies and natural health protocols have had a significant effect on Andrew's overall experience and ability to function in this life. Here's what has helped us the most:

Basic nutrition such as eating a natural, whole foods-based diet is foundational. Whole foods includes most anything nature provides in its whole form: fruit, vegetables, nuts, seeds and their oils (cold-pressed), fatty foods like avocado, olives, coconut and their oils/milk, whole grains, legumes, eggs, meat, poultry, fish. Even natural sugars are included: raw honey, maple syrup, coconut sugar. At present, we have the convenience of health foods that are made with natural, often whole food, ingredients including natural sugars—crackers, cookies, granola, breads, snacks. With health as a goal for the whole family, there is no room in the diet for processed foods, devoid of nutrients. This includes foods containing refined sugar. From there, we make sure to exclude all foods that contain artificial ingredients, especially food colours and flavours, artificial sweeteners, preservatives, MSG (and all forms of glutamate).

Quality food, grown in chemical-free environments and nutrient-rich soil, is important. We buy organic and/or local, as much as possible. We look for foods labelled non-GMO. We are aware of how pervasive the pesticide glyphosate is, so we avoid corn, soy, and sugar as much as possible. Andrew eats a gluten-free, dairy-free diet. When he does have gluten, we observe behaviour changes, mental fatigue ("dazed", appearing tired), and overnight bed-wetting.

In regards to gut-healing diets overall, we find Andrew does best on a paleo-type diet—one rich in fats, some animal protein, with plenty of vegetables, fruit and nuts. Andrew's most significant shift occurred when we committed to the "Gut and Psychology Syndrome" (GAPS) diet for six solid months: We saw textbook bowel movements, improved energy, mental clarity and processing, and more "presence". The GAPS diet, however, is a very prep-and cooking-intense program requiring a full commitment to achieve the best results. It is not where I suggest families begin! Building a healthy eating routine that is sustainable for the long-term, while perhaps adding in components of paleo (e.g., more vegetables) or "GAPS" (e.g., cooking with bone broths), is a great place to start.

We live in a world that is more toxic (with more "stressors") than ever before, and our food is less nutrient-rich (grown in nutrient-depleted soils, often with a sterile soil microbiome due to conventional farming practices and regular pesticide use, combined with long-transport nutrient loss, and over-processing of the foods and ingredients themselves)—we absolutely have a need for nutrient supplementation! Combine that with a sensory system that is heightened, our highly-sensitive children may experience more stress in their body-mind than others, creating an even greater need for supportive nutrients.

We created a simplified supplement list. Our priority nutrients include: vitamin D3 drops/spray, high-quality probiotic, whole food fruit, vegetable, berry concentrate, magnesium. Over the years, we have had a more extensive supplement list—especially during a committed gut-healing or detox protocol—but the foundational nutrients listed above have never changed.

Daily compliance is key for best results. We found a routine that was most successful for our family: supplements are taken at breakfast. For Andrew, this involves opening all capsules and emptying the powders into a small glass jar, adding a bit of unsweetened juice, shaking it up, drawing it into a plastic syringe, then shooting it into his mouth, lips pursed, followed by a "chaser" of something he likes—a true labour of love! When all goes well, it works, but it took three months of resistance before Andrew knew it wasn't going away. We have continued with this method now for eight years. I always know when we have gone off course with our routine as, within weeks, Andrew's behaviour is different—more tired, more irritable. I remind myself how worth it it is to commit.

We use supportive baths a few times a week, more specifically, an Epsom salt bath before bed. The magnesium sulfate in the salt has many benefits. Magnesium is calming to the body/nerves, and helps with anxiety and sleep. The sulfate acts as a precursor to one of the most potent and important antioxidants in the body: glutathione. Glutathione is essential for detoxification, immune system function, reducing/neutralizing free radicals, and preventing cellular damage and disease.

Clay baths are also excellent for detoxification (an alternative to chelation). They can be used weekly, for a period of consecutive months, but not ongoing. We used them under the advice of a functional medical doctor, though they are very safe. It is important to choose a high-quality, non contaminated, clinically proven magnetic clay product.

Brain-body movement is absolutely one of the most helpful therapies for Andrew was brain-body movement therapy. All body movements provide feedback to the brain, tracing neural pathways that get ingrained over time. Brain-body therapy encouraged Andrew to move his body in a way that not only increased his coordination and body awareness, but nourished new pathways in his brain that brought him calm, happiness, and more clarity and presence. He can climb play structures, ride a bike, and learn new body routines (such as brushing teeth, making a snack) because of this brain-body integration.

Homeopathy has also been hugely helpful, as has energy work (e.g., cranial-sacral, osteopathy, energetic healing) and other holistic therapies along the way. They have all contributed to Andrew's success. They led us to where we are today. I believe that they are an essential piece of the picture. But it wasn't about just that—for us, anyway. It was about much more than that. It was about the subtleties: the stuff you can't find in books, or online, or from "the experts". It was about the stuff you'd miss if you weren't looking. Stuff you'd miss if you weren't paying attention. Stuff you can only learn by living it. It was about opening our eyes. About living in our heart. And it was about learning to trust our gut. This is what led us to the single most impactful tool that has changed the course of our life for our family, and most certainly for Andrew, Spelling to Communicate.

Spelling to Communicate (S2C) is an education and alternative and augmentative communication (AAC) system involving a "Speller" (typically a non-speaking, minimally-speaking, or unreliably-speaking person), the use of a physical letterboard (stencil or laminate) with a trained and trusted communication and regulation partner (CRP—often a parent, close friend or teacher, and/or S2C practitioner). The method involves regular practice on the letter boards with the Speller and partner, building trust, skill, accuracy, and fluency.

It doesn't always come easy. It took us months and months, with hundreds of hours of practice to fine-tune the physical act (the brain-motor path) of holding a pencil, then getting Andrew's brain to coordinate his body to move his arm to point (poke) the precise letter that he wants on the letterboard with the pencil in his hand. Eventually, it can lead to independent typing on a keyboard, but that is a huge motor planning feat. As a pair, we go through "topic lessons" that get Andrew (the Speller) to practice and fine-tune the physical act (motor path) of pointing to letters to spell words to communicate. Words lead to sentences which leads to opening up a whole world of expression, communication, and possibility with your child.

In its simplest form, Spelling to Communicate teaches individuals with motor challenges the purposeful motor skills necessary to point to letters to spell as an alternative means of communication (AAC). The goal is to achieve synchronicity between the brain and body. Skilled and rigorously trained communication partners teach purposeful motor skills using a hierarchy of verbal and gestural prompts. As motor skills improve through consistent practice, students progress from pointing to letters on letterboards to spell, to typing on a keyboard. Accordingly, communication output moves from concrete to abstract as motor skills progress.

Did I think my child knew the alphabet? Sure, maybe. Did I think he could spell? No, not words like arachnid and endocrinology! Or simple words, either. Did I think my child was as smart (cognitively able) as he is? I had no idea.

But we need to give our autistic children more credit! They have been observing text and hearing it in context their whole lives. We need to presume competence. And we need to get ready for what they have to say, for they have been waiting a long time to say it. This method of communication has changed everything. And the truth is, we weren't looking for it.

But I knew there was more for us, for Andrew—I could see it in my child's eyes, beyond his eyes. I didn't know how to access it. I didn't know how to get it out, but I knew it was all there. And in one of the darkest nights of our journey, where there was no light, only dark, I looked at my husband with tears in my eyes and a certainty I'd never known before and declared: *I will never give up on that child.* Never. Not ever. I will keep looking, keep digging, and hoping—because *I know* there is more—for him and for us.

No stone left unturned.

I like to say "it found us". And the rest is history, though in many ways, it feels like it's only just beginning. Admittedly, it's been a tough road. On paper, I'm not sure I would have chosen this story: you will have a child who doesn't speak. Who walks a unique path. Who doesn't come with "answers". Not in the way that you expect them. As a mother, you will be stripped down to your bare bones—raw, torn, broken. You will wonder how you will ever get up again.

But our children teach us what we need to learn. My children have taught me my strength, my character, my courage.

We all have our story. In many ways, ours is a story of perseverance, of resilience. And certainly one of trust. What could have been a story of giving up, became a story of purpose. What once felt like a life sentence, became a new beginning.

About two years into the method, I sat with Andrew. It was Christmas, and after writing out messages, letter by letter, for his teachers, friends and family. I asked if he would like to write a message to his mom, to me. This might seem funny or forward, but sometimes, initiation is tricky for Andrew. So even though he might want to do or "say" something—even if he has already been thinking about it—his body won't follow through and initiate on his behalf. He answered, "Yes".

And as I watched each letter, his words, unfold in front of me, I felt a wave wash over me—like every single moment that led up to this point washed right over me, bringing me to this exact present moment in time. My breath escaped me as I read:

Mom
Feeling overcome with a beautiful feeling
of love and gratitude for you
and all you have done for me
all these years
I am forever grateful.
How you had the patience and perseverance
is a gift I will keep close in my heart always
Here's to so much ahead for us.

Speechless. Moved to tears. Silent streams down my cheeks. Every single moment in life brings you to exactly where you are. And where you are meant to be.

My dear sweet boy.

What you have given me over these years, and in this moment, is a gift that is, ironically, hard to put into words. Personal insight and opportunities for growth that many people search a lifetime for. If I tried to recount what the lessons were—what the learning has been—it would be pages. But if I look back, even before my life with children, these are the lessons that showed up, as they do, over and over and over:

Accept. Accept that life will look different than you expect. Accept that there will be pain, and sadness, and challenge, and tons and tons of joy if you can see it. Be open. Be open to a life that takes you in a direction you can't predict, or that you didn't know existed. One you certainly can't control. Trust. Trust in the process of life. In the journey of living. And live it. That's all you need to do.

We don't know what lies ahead. I get overwhelmed thinking about it. For me, it's horrible not to know. But if there's one thing I've learned, it's to pay attention to the lessons:

To accept,

to be open,

and to trust.

All things lead you to exactly where you are meant to be.

—Susan Baker

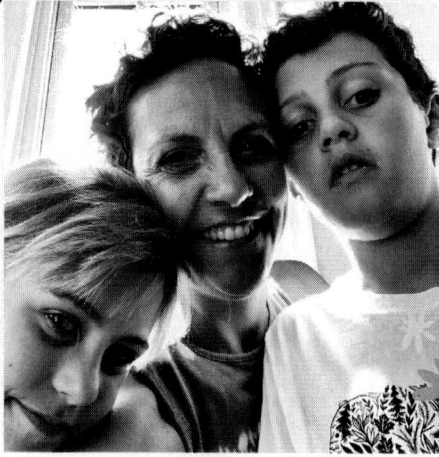

Susan Baker

Susan Baker is the mom to two beautiful children, Andrew, 12, and Abby, 8, at the time of this writing. She is a holistic nutritionist and has been in the natural health industry since 2001. She is the author of *Life, Love & Autism*, an online blog that chronicles their family's journey of growth and challenge, including love, loss and an autism diagnosis. She lives in Toronto, Ontario with her husband and children. She continues to inspire health in others through her online programs and social media presence. "*Life, Love & Autism* has become a beautiful 'documentation' of our life as a family. Often hilarious, sometimes hard, but most certainly, inspiring, *Life, Love & Autism* is raw and real, my heart on my sleeve. The blog is way beyond autism: it is about the human connection, and what brings us together. It is about the joy, the challenge, and the learning that comes from it all. And it is as much for me as it is for you. A journey—lived, documented, and shared." —Susan

Email: susan@behealthyforlife.ca
Blog: Search *Life, Love & Autism* on Facebook and Instagram
Website: www.lifeloveautism.com

Fruit & vegetable concentrate (in capsules, chewables):
https://sb23470.canada.juiceplus.com

Ollie's Story—From Nonna's Heart

By Lia Bandola

September 14th, 2019

This is the day that our world changed forever—the day that our world got turned upside down. The day our beautiful Oliver James Shearer was born. It was a miraculous day and so joyful in the beginning. Dana (my daughter and Ollie's mom) had an uneventful and generally great pregnancy. This was her first pregnancy and as she is a researcher by profession she treated this the same as she does her work. Lots of reading and research. She did all the right things and all her health visits and ultrasounds showed that everything was great.

Her water broke in the evening of the 13th and they went to Markham-Stouffville hospital where her midwife team would meet her. Her delivery was also as perfect as it could be and she brought Ollie into the world with minimal pushing. I was there to witness this blessed event, as was her husband, Kyle. Dana's team of midwives were fantastic and they also felt all went extremely well. When Ollie came out he was quite blue and very still. The cord had been loosely around his neck but the midwives felt it did not cut off any oxygen. He did quickly come around and was pinking up and moving soon after, so it was felt that all was well.

All of Ollie's vitals were good and he appeared to be healthy. He weighed 5 lbs. 6 oz. and was three weeks early. A little small, but otherwise seemed good. I was over the moon in love and filled with joy. I was so happy and excited for my daughter and son-in-law, Kyle to be embarking on their journey into parenthood.

The usual round of congratulations, phone calls, and well wishes almost immediately started to come in—the beauty of Social Media. My husband came and Kyle's mom also arrived shortly after. As we were getting a chance to get to see and hold Ollie, he started to have a few "blue" episodes. He would stop breathing briefly and turn a greyish-blue. This of course caused us some alarm, but they were very short episodes and when we pointed it out to the midwife doing his chart and records, she was not concerned and said it was "normal" to see this sometimes in small, premature babies. Ollie was just on the cusp of being considered a preemie—Dana went into labour 1 day before the 37 week mark, so they were putting him in that category.

Still no real concerns. Then the next day they told us they heard a heart murmur and wanted to explore further with an ECG. A paediatric cardiologist came into the room with the ECG machine, hooked Ollie up and that's when she saw the large hole in his heart. At that point, she felt it was not so large that it was inevitable that he would need surgery to close it up. However, we would later learn that, in fact, he would need surgery as it was considered to be a large hole. More on that later, because as it turned out, that certainly was not the worst of his issues.

It was in the aftercare ward, where Dana and Ollie had been moved to, that the nurses seemed more concerned about the blue episodes, but said they couldn't really gauge it without having seen it. Fortunately, Dana and Ollie were kept longer than originally planned because Ollie needed an extra blood test to monitor his jaundice levels. A nurse came in to help Dana with latching late Sunday evening and Ollie had a blue episode and she saw it. She quickly got him down to the NICU and had him checked out by a paediatrician who felt this was definitely something of concern and needed to be explored further. And that's when the real journey began.

They brought in a team from SickKids to transport Ollie to their hospital where they could do a full neurological workup to determine why he was having these episodes. My husband and I were home sleeping and we got that dreaded middle of the night call. Kyle told us they were taking Ollie to SickKids by ambulance and they needed a ride there because, of course, neither he nor Dana were in any condition to drive. They had been up virtually for 54 hours at this point and were in shock at the turn of the events.

Gary and I threw on some clothes and raced to the hospital. We were allowed to go in and say goodbye to Ollie. That moment was one of the most devastating moments for me—so far at that point—because we would see a whole lot worse with him. He was hooked up to all kinds of monitors and apparatus in the incubator they would transport him in. He was heavily sedated and was so still. I tried so hard to hold it together because I didn't want to add to Dana and Kyle's alarm. So I swallowed hard, shed a few tears and said to myself "stay strong" for Dana and Kyle.

Off we went to SickKids—the first of many, many journeys there. Silence in the car, I encouraged Dana and Kyle to close their eyes for a bit. They did but no one actually slept. My mind was racing. What was going to happen to Ollie. Would he live? Would he have some kind of brain damage? Neurological issues? I couldn't stop the horrible thoughts running through my mind.

On a side note, I am a cognitive behaviour therapist, general counsellor, and life coach. I have had years and years of training. I have counselled and coached hundreds of people and helped them to make great changes in their lives, and in their mental and emotional states. But in that moment, I was just a scared, devastated grandmother watching her daughter suffering like never before. I felt helpless, confused, worried and a whole gamut of emotions that all the training and experience in the world was not going to help. In that moment, I felt like my world had stopped on its axis.

We arrived at SickKids and headed up to the NICU. Ollie had arrived with the team and they were starting the barrage of tests, including blood tests, CT scan, and other tests. Later, an MRI was scheduled. We sat in the waiting room. Other parents were in there. There was an eery quiet, except for odd crying sounds or groans. It still haunts me to this day. I believe I do have some PTSD from it, and whenever I go by that room (which I have many times) I still get a pang in my chest and feel like I can't breathe.

At this point, Dana and Kyle are finally able to go see their son. Doctors talked to them and told them there were more tests to be done and it would be best for them to go get some sleep while we waited for results to come in. Bear in mind that Dana had only given birth less than 60 hours before and she needed to get some rest for her own healing. Reluctantly, we all went home.

The next morning, we went back to the hospital. Again, Gary and I drove Dana and Kyle. My husband is a rock and he was the safest driver at that point. At the hospital Dana and Kyle went in to see Ollie to get an update. Time starts to get fuzzy at this point for me. I do remember them coming out and giving us the devastating news that Ollie had a brain abnormality. He is missing the Corpus Callosum which is the bundle of nerves between the left and right sides of the brain that mainly does the signalling from one side to the other.

Fear again gripped me. What did this mean? Would he be able to function? Can you live without it? So many questions, and so much terror. But again, my main concern was for my daughter. "Hold it together" I told myself once again. I hugged my girl and told her it would all be alright—even though I didn't really know that. I had to make her believe that.

Then the round of many phone calls to be made to family. Having to tell my sons and their partners was so hard. Again, I just went into protective mom-mode and told them it would be OK. We just needed to be strong for Dana and Kyle and be a good support for them. Inside I was crumbling, though.

We now knew Ollie had a congenital heart defect and a brain abnormality. And the "why" questions started. As I said, Dana had a very healthy pregnancy—she did all the right things. She had multiple ultrasounds, regular prenatal visits and tests. All seemed perfect. How did two such significant defects not get caught?

The research started. Fortunately, my niece has her PhD in neuroscience and has done years of research in childhood brain disorders. Of course, she was one of the first people I called. That conversation brought me great comfort as she explained that because infants' brains are so pliable and still developing, there was a good chance Ollie's brain would compensate for the deficit and he could potentially have no developmental issues. Or if he did, we could get early intervention in and he could overcome any delays he may have. By now my head was spinning! Processing the heart defect, the brain deficit, what this could mean for Ollie's quality of life, what this would mean for Dana and Kyle as parents. It all started to feel like too much, too fast.

Because Ollie now had two abnormalities that we knew of, there was some suspicion in the doctors' minds that it could be as a result of a genetic abnormality. So they took blood from Ollie to send to genetics and Dana and Kyle also had to submit blood samples. That would be a pretty long wait though for results. So in the meantime, the concern was to keep Ollie stabilized and monitor his vitals and heart functioning.

He was started on medications for his heart and watched closely. In the meantime, Dana was pumping her breast milk and it was being given to Ollie by bottle. He had difficulty suckling right from the start so they were giving him other fluids to make sure he was not becoming dehydrated. He was stable and the barrage of tests were completed. After eight days in the NICU at SickKids, it was decided that Ollie was stable and they had done all they could do at this point for him there. So they felt he could be moved to a Level 2 NICU (SickKids is a level four—the highest) and they just needed to find a bed at a hospital closer to home. He was moved to Lakeridge Health in Oshawa. We were so happy because he was stable enough to move there and because he was closer to all of us making it much easier to visit and be with Dana.

That is when the rollercoaster really became crazy! First day there, the neonatologist came in after he had checked Ollie out and conferred with the SickKids doctors and told us that results of the Infant Screening Test (all newborns in Ontario get this test at birth) showed positive results for the possibility of Cystic Fibrosis. Another kick in the gut. The doctor reassured us this did not mean he had it—just that a marker had come up. We would have to wait to get more tests done. After finally doing multiple tests, it was determined that Ollie was a carrier for CF so this was some good news really as he does not have the disease but will have to just be aware of that down the road if he does decide to have children.

Day three at Lakeridge NICU brought the next terrifying situation. Ollie's heart rate sky-rocketed and he had what is called an SVT (supraventricular tachycardia) event. I had just arrived at the hospital and went to buzz in when I heard the call for docs to get to the NICU, saw a flurry of people running into the NICU and was told to wait outside. My stomach churned, my heart started racing, and while I prayed it wasn't Ollie, my intuition told me it was.

Finally, someone came out and told me it was in fact Ollie and he had a team in there with him. I asked to be allowed in to be with my daughter because I knew she must be terrified and needed my support. She had sent Kyle home to get some things done, they had just moved into their new home one week prior to Ollie making his early entrance. They finally allowed me to go in, and of course, Dana was distraught and happy I was there. Here we go again, I thought. "Suck it up and hold it together" I told myself yet again.

We got Kyle back there as his mother drove him there. He took over for me when he got there. I didn't want to leave but had to—only two people allowed in there at a time. I took a last glance at what seemed like frenzied activity by all kinds of medical personnel. Monitors being hooked up, echocardiogram being done, IVs put in, incubator brought in; organized chaos was what it felt like.

I went out and waited in the waiting room with Kyle's mom for hours—literally. It was torture to not know what was happening. Was Ollie okay? Was Dana okay? My emotions and concern were heightened for my grandson and my daughter. But I stayed calm, kept reassuring Patricia, Kyle's mom, that he would be okay. There I go again—being the support for everyone around me. And inside I was screaming! Finally, Dana and Kyle came out looking grim but also calm. They had stabilized Ollie and his heart rate had normalized. More medication to keep it that way. More questions. Is this related to his heart defect? We are told no. Completely unrelated! How is that possible? Everyone is exhausted. We all go home and try to get some rest. By now, it's after 9 p.m. I was there since noon. Little food and a lot of anxiety. This would be a pattern that would ensue over the next several months.

Day four at Lakeridge—the rollercoaster takes a major dive. I picked Dana up and we headed to the hospital. Kyle had decided to go in to work as he was supposed to start a new job and there was training he needed to get to. Since Ollie was stable, he thought it would be okay to go in. He was close to the hospital and just a phone call away. Good thing, because that's when the biggest crisis hit.

Ollie had rallied from his heart episode the day before and was trying to eat from the bottle but when we got there the nurse said he had been spitting up a lot. Also, she said he had a slight fever and gave him some baby Tylenol, so maybe it was that. But they were watching him closely. They were bringing in the neonatologist to check him out. In the meantime, Dana was doing some skin-to-skin with Ollie and he threw up all over her. There was a shift change with the nurses and the new nurse came over and looked at Ollie and the colour of his spit up and suddenly went into action. She didn't like the colour and said there was bile and his fever had increased. His belly was quickly distending and he was in visible pain–moaning and wincing. An image I will never get out of my head. He was already on Tylenol but she upped the dose, got him on antibiotics, and got the doctor in right away. After he checked him over, he confirmed her suspicions and concerns. Ollie may have perforated bowels and could be toxic. We needed to get him back to SickKids as soon as possible. A team from SickKids was brought in—an even bigger team this time. They checked him over and did an ultrasound and confirmed that Ollie in fact had NEC (necrotizing enterocolitis) a very serious disease affecting a newborn's intestines.

Once they felt Ollie was stable enough to move, they transported him again to SickKids for more extensive testing and diagnostics. And, once again, we made the long trek back to SickKids where we waited for results of further tests and diagnosis. The doctors did confirm NEC and said they were unsure of the extent of the disease so wanted to just keep a close monitor of him overnight. They again told us to all go home and get some rest. We did.

Early in the morning, we again got a distressing call. Dana and Kyle were called by SickKids and told that Ollie had gotten worse in the night and they were doing emergency surgery as soon as possible and to get to the hospital quickly. Yet again, we threw on our clothes and drove Ollie's parents to SickKids. Another silent, anxiety-ridden ride.

When we arrived, they were getting Ollie ready to be taken to surgery. They gave us all the information about the surgery and told us where to wait.

And then the agony of the waiting began. The surgery was over five hours. The doctor took Dana and Kyle into a private room when they finished. The rest of us waited.

After the surgeon left them, Dana and Kyle shared what he told them. They did need to remove 50% of Ollie's lower intestine because it was so badly diseased. The good news was that his upper intestine was virtually unaffected and they didn't have to do anything surgically there. We were relieved and simultaneously still very concerned. They said the next 24 hours would be critical. We were still dealing with a life and death situation. Those words were devastating to hear.

Ollie had a colostomy bag because they had to remove so much of his bowel, but they told us that if he healed well, they could re-attach the colon to the rectum in a few months. Ollie was in the NICU for almost two months at this point. When they felt he had healed well enough they moved him to a room where Dana could stay with him. This was the first of three "hotel" stays Dana would have with Ollie at SickKids. Ollie was released a week later and he was finally able to go home for the first time since he was born. That was a happy day!

The next few months were all about getting Ollie healed and growing. That was an issue. He was not putting enough weight on and the decision was made to put the NG feeding tube back in to make sure he was getting enough milk. Dana was still pumping and supplementing her breastmilk with formula. Ollie started to put some weight on.

They booked his bowel reattachment surgery for December 13th. Again, back at SickKids for the second surgery. And again, the waiting and anxiety, though this time was different. It was not emergency surgery. There was a very positive outcome expected and the surgeon was very confident that all would go well and Ollie would once again have a fully functioning gastric system. And he did! I was overjoyed for Dana and Kyle. What started as a terrifying crisis had ended with the best outcome we could expect.

By this time, Ollie had become a bit of a celebrity. We are blessed to have so many wonderful family and friends that became Ollie's cheerleaders and Dana and Kyle's supporters. I reached out on social media for prayers and healing, positive energy to be sent for Ollie. I was overwhelmed at the enormous support that we had. Literally hundreds of people, some that I knew well and some that I didn't even know. There were so many generous offers of help in so many ways. I was so touched by this outpouring of love and generosity. And that became my salvation; where I could allow my real emotions to be expressed, even if it was sitting by myself reading all the beautiful comments, sobbing, and letting the emotions flow.

Our strong warrior healed extremely fast from this surgery and two days before Christmas, Ollie was back home. The best Christmas present ever! We enjoyed the holidays immensely with Ollie as part of the festivities. Once the holidays were over though, I had my crash. Things had settled down for now with Ollie. Dana and Kyle were adjusting to their new life with Ollie and I was alone more than I had been for months. I got very ill—a bout of bronchitis that had started at the end of November but I think I held it all together—as I kept telling myself, even physically because of the surgery coming up and the many trips to the hospital that we were making outside of the surgeries for follow-ups, testing for other possible issues, ophthalmology, hearing tests, motor skills, CF testing, pre-op tests, and more. SickKids became our second home. I always went with Dana because Kyle had to get back to work. He had exhausted all holidays, lieu time and sick time he had coming to him.

By the time the holidays were over and I didn't need to be "on" as much, my body and mind said "Okay, it's time!" I was exhausted, mentally and physically. I became depressed and the sadness just overtook me. I did manage to reach into my "toolbox" though, and started getting back to some of my healthy practices that I had virtually let go of since Ollie was born. I took time to meditate, journal, do some yoga, get out for some walks, and was able to give myself some care. I cried a lot, got angry, did the "why us?" thing and just let myself feel whatever was coming up that I had buried for months. At the end of a few weeks, I started to feel better. I saw my chiropractor, got some massages, and just generally got back to my self-care. I realized that I could be an even better support for Dana if I took care of myself first.

In January we got the genetic testing results. Turns out Ollie has a rare chromosomal abnormality. He is missing a section from Chromosome 1 and has an extra piece on Chromosome 11. The geneticists we met with said they have never seen this particular combination and there are literally no research journals on this. Their best guess is that Ollie's particular defects are as a result of the missing piece on Chromosome 1, as they have seen those issues before related to that abnormality. This is an inherited genetic abnormality. So, we now had some answers as to why.

Fast forward to February. Ollie needed to have his heart repaired sooner rather than later. He was starting to show signs that his heart was working too hard with the large hole and it was affecting his eating and growth. He got booked for surgery for February 10th, but suddenly Dana got a call on Monday the 3rd saying there was a cancellation and could she get Ollie down the next day for surgery. Of course, they said yes, and at 5 a.m. the next morning, we were heading down to SickKids yet again for surgery.

This time, for some reason, I had a terrible sense of foreboding. Maybe because it was open heart surgery. My mom had open heart surgery in her mid-70s and perhaps it brought back some memories there. Not sure why, but my usual positive thoughts had a lot more worry in them.

When we got to the hospital this time, there were all the pre-op tests and preparation. Then every single member of the surgical team came in to talk to us. They were so reassuring and confident that we were all put at ease—well, somewhat. It was much harder this time watching Ollie getting taken into the surgical area. He was now more engaging and smiling and my heart was aching seeing him go. Again, the routine of waiting and waiting which by now had become kind of familiar, and in a strange way, a little easier.

The surgery went extremely well and they were able to repair all the issues—large hole, smaller hole and a couple of other small repairs. We were elated and I just knew in my heart that Ollie would make a full recovery.

And he has! Today he is thriving, growing, engaging, no signs of any significant motor delays and is starting to eat better by the bottle. He even started on solid foods recently! There are still some unknowns. Some possibilities of delays in speech, learning, and large motor skills. But we are so blessed to live where we do, where there are already many community and developmental supports in place. Ollie is surrounded by so many people who love him and who will help him with whatever he needs.

Nonna—I'm doing so much better, too, seeing my daughter being able to just do regular mom-things with Ollie. Seeing her happier and more confident. Being able to get out and enjoy time with her friends and husband–Nonna will babysit any time! And there are lots of other people who will gladly take over from Nonna.

I know this story has a much longer way to go, but for now we are enjoying every little bit of progress we see Ollie make, enjoying his already fun personality and just loving and watching our beautiful Ollie grow and flourish.

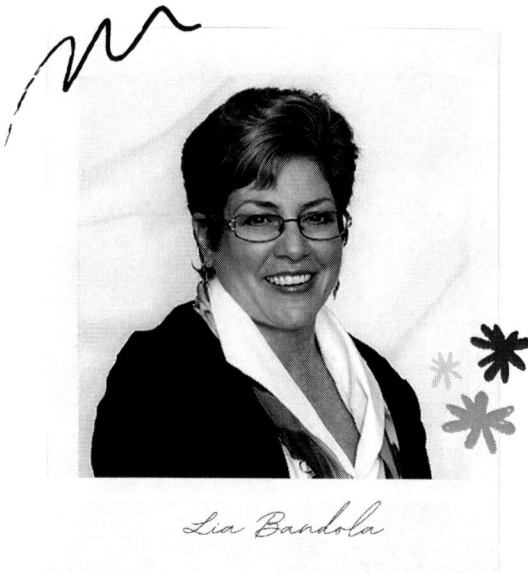

Lia Bandola

Lia has been married for almost 42 years to Gary, mom to three grown children—Aaron, Kevin, and Dana and grandmother "Nonna" to three beautiful grandsons—Nathan, Rylan, and Ollie. Lia is the owner of Life Lessons Unlimited providing personal coaching and counselling services, including group programs. She works with people to uncover possible hidden traumas, thought patterns and behaviours that may be keeping them stuck and feeling like they are just "surviving". She then provides the tools to change their patterns so they can move forward to create a life where they are truly thriving. Lia is a registered social service worker, cognitive behaviour therapist, certified life skills coach, a certified true colours trainer, and is in the process of becoming a certified professional empowerment coach. She is a published author, professional speaker, workshop facilitator, and works with individuals, couples, families and groups.

Website: www.lifelessons.ca
Facebook: @lifelessonsunlimited
Instagram: @butterflylessons.

If you go to her website, you will be able to access her free home study program called _Courage, Risks and Rewards_.

Lia's Publications include:

Chapter: "I Can Have it All, Can't I? Overcoming the Superwoman Trap!" in *Expert Women Who Speak, Speak Out*, Vol. 5, Editors Adele Alfano and Kathy Glover Scott, 2005

The Power of Women United, Confidence Born of Strength and Wisdom, The Ultimate Publishing House, 2009—a Canadian Best Seller

So, Your Child Has Autism...

By Cheryl Benitah

> *"Jack? Can you look at me? Look over here
> Jack." The doctor snapped his fingers
> making a futile attempt to get my son's
> attention. "Okay, he has autism. Get on the
> waitlist and google Autism Ontario."*

That's it. That's what we got. Two sentences that sucker punched us and left my husband and I in a muted trance. To this day, I have no recollection of leaving the doctor's office or the next several hours that followed. The only thought I can remember having was 'what now, where are the instructions, is there a pamphlet?'

With 20 years in the field of child and youth counselling under my belt and two spirited daughters in tow, I was not new to motherhood. Third time's a charm…

I entirely miscalculated the metamorphosis Jack's arrival would set in motion. Life with Jack is comparable to a scene from the movie *Fast and Furious* on fast forward with unexpected pit stops to take in the sites.

The next four years proved to be a complete immersion in the culture of being an autism mom. As I look back and reflect on the journey this far, I feel overwhelmed. There are so many more years to go. I can't help but question my longevity. It's a scary thought. Having no point of reference or compass to lead the way is like being thrown into unchartered waters with no life raft for a religious planner like myself. What can I expect life to be like from this point forward? There are no clear answers to that or any questions I may have. The truth is, whenever I think I have adequately prepared for any and all possible hurdles, I get propelled backwards like an elastic band snapping back in my face. The only planning left is to have no plan at all.

I can clearly recall distinct moments of consciousness that I now know were essential in navigating through the impromptu adventure ahead. Everyone's journey is unique. No two stories are ever comparable when you are the one living it. The content is very individual, but I have come to find that many, if not all, autism families experience the same rite of passage.

Guilt

The first real emotion I felt for a long time was guilt. I was flooded with responsibility and shame. I scoured my brain for all the reasons I was responsible. What did I do? What didn't I do? Was it the occasional missed prenatal vitamins, or maybe satisfying my craving for blue cheese and salami sandwiches that I had convinced myself were insignificant in comparison to the countless weeks of an appetite gone AWOL? Ultimately, it didn't really matter which misdeed caused it. The weight of failing my little boy was crushing. I never said the words out loud. I punished myself far more than any other person would and was petrified at the thought of someone agreeing with me. No amount of encouraging words or supportive embraces could erase the immeasurable blame I had assigned myself.

It was a long time before I came to accept that the guilt was less about placing blame and more about replenishing control over a situation that I knew couldn't be 'fixed'. My self-inflicted penance was a scapegoat from accepting what I already knew to be true. If I was to blame, if eating soft cheeses and uncured meat were remotely at fault, knowing that wouldn't change any of it. I needed a minute to feel sorry for myself before I was able to forgive myself for any fault I may have had.

Grief

Possibly this is the most numbing response I have experienced. The sense of loss is unending. Yes, I have a beautiful, healthy little boy. I am very mindful of how blessed I am. That doesn't discredit my right to mourn the loss of what was to be.

Like any parent does when they learn of a new arrival, I had instinctively projected my hopes and dreams for my little one's entire existence. It's human nature. I envisioned each milestone: his first step, graduation day, his wedding, even as far as the cool Nanna I plan to be! My heart was flooded with sorrow. The picture I had painted for my sweet boy instantly faded into a muddled blur when handed that diagnosis letter. I wholeheartedly expect that Jack will be just fine. Jack will be great. I truly believe that. I believe in Jack. I am, however, not naïve enough to think it will come easy or without shedding much blood, sweat, and tears.

So yes, I'm entitled to grieve. I don't think I will ever completely stop. Every milestone will be a reminder. When you are told how lucky you are that he doesn't cry for you in the middle of the night, your heart aches to be needed.

Wondering if you will ever hear your child's voice leaves a void that eats away at you. Silently hoping that he will experience the joy and bond that siblings share while watching my nephew, two years younger, squeal in delight while playing with my daughters.

Grief is healing and necessary for the soul. It allows me to move past the picture I envisioned and embrace the masterpiece that Jack chooses to create.

Becoming a special needs family is not a simple amendment of social status. I would have never predicted what a significant undertaking it is. Depending on the degree of severity of diagnosis or child's needs, it could entail a complete transformation of lifestyle. Our idea of what would have to change typically revolved around Jack. Before him, we were never the type of parents to schedule our lives around nap times or temper tantrums. Of course, we anticipated some tweaking, but it would have never occurred to us that continual change would be our new constant. You might recall me mentioning my incessant need to plan—autism is a planner's *kryptonite*. Jack is forever evolving, which means his tolerances, likes, dislikes, and sensitivities can change as frequently as daily. Add the nonverbal element to the equation and I often feel powerless when it comes to anticipating how he will react to any given situation or social event we attend.

Jack's needs are just the tip of the iceberg when considering what each outing may bring about. Aside from weighing the value of each event, we also must factor in whether it is suitable for all attending. Should my daughters accompany their brother to every autism-related event? Is it fair to them? No, just as it wouldn't make sense to have Jack attend his sisters eight hour taekwondo tournament or gymnastics meet. Accommodations must be made for each member of the family. This is typically an easy adjustment as it benefits all involved. A more delicate shift is when dealing with friends and families and the endless birthday parties, holidays, and all the other various events where attendance is typically implied. No matter how supportive your circle is, *no one* will ever truly get it. The truth is that unless you are on the receiving end of our day-to-day existence, you couldn't possibly truly appreciate why missing a birthday dinner or wanting to spend a holiday at home alone is the best decision for all involved.

I am thankful for the assurances that it will be fine, but I also am hopeful that one can entrust me to do what's best for my family and unfortunately that doesn't always work in everyone's favor. That being said, it's important not to isolate yourself from those that care about you. People may not always say or do all the right things but their intentions are generally good. This journey is a whirlwind of ups and downs and can feel very lonely, maintaining healthy and positive relationships are of essential value. Communication is key, express your concerns or needs, invite questions, share setbacks and triumphs, accept help when it is offered and be clear about what is helpful if you have to ask for it. Many won't be up to the task and your circle will get smaller which is okay, because superficial ties will require invaluable time and energy better spent elsewhere.

Acceptance and empathy are a requirement and should be given freely without any obligation to justify or seek approval. Establishing honest communication, empathy, and understanding within your circle will be of benefit to everyone.

Opinions

Everyone has one. I smiled and nodded as I half listened to someone recount how great the autistic guy turned out in *The Good Docto*r, all the while envisioning slugging them in the head with Jack's PEC binder. So often, people who have nothing to say satisfy their own needs by saying *anything*.

"Have you tried going gluten free; dairy free, dye free, sugar free? I hear it's good for autism". – *Why yes, I may even try starving autism out of him.*

"Well you're lucky he isn't aggressive" —*but his mother can be!*

"He doesn't look autistic"—*Oh, no? Well, it must be the way we parted his hair today.*

They just keep coming and even when I think I've heard the worst of it, some guy who met you no longer than 30 seconds ago will hurl a curveball at you, suggesting what sounds an awful lot like waterboarding, insisting that you can "flush out the autism with water". No witty return could have matched that priceless nugget of wisdom. Mind… blown!

Most of the unsolicited advice is simply laughable or ill-advised. Comic relief at best for the next coffee date with your fellow autism mamas. I won't pretend that it isn't exasperating to be imparted with typecast autism clichés. I've been held captive to countless tales of the time someone met someone with autism which qualifies them to have an opinion and that I would be remiss not to take notes. It happens so often that I actively avoid most social settings that are likely not attended by other autism families. All that aside, I can also empathize with one's sense of duty to relate when sharing the news of a diagnosis.

Ultimately, no matter how indifferent I am to the opinions of others or how amusing I find one's reaction to an equally ridiculous response, I'm compelled to model behaviour I expect my children to adopt when inevitably facing these circumstances. I do my best to approach every situation objectively. After all, my sharp tongue and zero filter has made me no stranger to "foot-in-mouth syndrome". Taking into consideration the person offering the advice and our relationship, most often, I find a smile and a nod to be the least engaging.

Don't get me wrong, there will be moments that will enrage you, break your heart, or have you seeking refuge for the inevitable "ugly cry". There will be the moments that will render you speechless as you fear for your child's future among the ones who have you questioning your faith in humanity. When a "devout and Godly" woman expressly interrupts your otherwise pleasant mother-and-son lunch date to advise you to "pray to God to make him *normal*". In these moments, you're overcome with a profound sense of sadness, your mind is flooded with emotions, and you're left numb. You dig deep, searching desperately for tolerance and the strength to stay composed. How could someone be so willfully ignorant? So many feel it is their right to impart personal beliefs, true or otherwise, onto others with no regard or accountability for the harm they cause. You can't possibly let this person walk away unaware of their twisted principles—and that's when you realize how stuck you are as a parent. On one hand, you feel justified in lashing out, obligated even, but understanding the depth of ignorance you are dealing with, you quickly accept that your wrath will not be received as warranted and will likely leave you feeling defeated.

On this day, my instinctual response shifted from a place of anger to feeling compelled to educate, not so much to her benefit but to hopefully spare a fellow parent she may feel the need to advise from having a similar encounter. Most importantly, for my son and every other individual on the spectrum at the mercy of such ill-informed individuals. That day, I surprised myself. I made a difference. I sparked change and it was empowering. I prompted reflection, albeit marginal, in the grand scheme of things, but movement nonetheless.

Team Jack Jack is composed of several star players. Whether presently in our circle or a past connection, each person has contributed towards Jack's development. When I first heard the term "building a team", I'll admit, I didn't quite buy into the idea. The only teammate I had was my husband. It's a nice gesture and sure, there were well-wishers and the instinctive look of commiseration that came with sharing the news of a diagnosis. At the end of the day, Serge and I would shoulder complete accountability for our son's quality of life.

Assuming that role is quite daunting and as I now understand, not necessary. Of course, as parents we are the primary caregivers, much like "team captains" and it is our privilege to handpick everyone that plays a part in Jack's journey. The people you surround yourself with fill in the gaps forming a solid unit. Each team is specific to the child but should consist of individuals who are unquestionably invested in their success. How do they engage your child? Is there a connection? What are their ethics? Do they align with your own? Most importantly, how does your child respond to them? After all, it's all about them. It's not a one size fits all situation and you are not bound to any one person. You know your child best, so take their cue. There will be times where you need to separate your needs from what's best for your child. So, you don't get the warm and fuzzies from one of the therapists, but they are effective and produce results. Which is of more value?

It's not a minor task. You won't always get it right and that can set you back. It's temporary, though, and a good reminder to establish appropriate boundaries. Becoming attached is understandable and may feel reassuring. I still cherish the memory of shedding tears alongside Jack's speech therapist as he spoke his first word. Experiencing this momentous milestone was as rewarding to her as it was to me. It's not unusual to feel comforted by someone who cares for your child. It can also cloud your judgement or hinder your ability to address concerns to avoid a fallout. If you do have to address something, don't make it personal, stick to the facts. Pay attention to the tone of the response and actions that follow. Did they acknowledge your concern? Did you feel heard? If necessary, were changes made? Were you involved in discussions/plans/changes regarding the issue? The outcome should instill a sense of resolve and ultimately be of benefit to your child.

If you feel uncomfortable talking to the people you leave your child with, it's probably time to re-evaluate what your expectations are, and possibly move on. Don't lose sight of the main objective. What is in the best interest of your child? Every decision should be made with that in mind. I consider myself to generally be a good judge of character and have made genuine connections with several of Jack's providers. Some that unfortunately left me disheartened and hurt more than I expected. It also served as a reminder to remain vigilant when making decisions on behalf of Jack, that they in fact are choices which ultimately benefit him.

As I learn to separate my role as Jack's advocate from being his mom, I feel more confident in my ability to balance wearing both hats. Having help from my own carefully devised team of a select few to lean on, vent with, listen to and let down my guard with has been essential. Never underestimate the value of commiseration and camaraderie between you and a fellow autism mama or papa.

When a solid team is composed, you feel lighter. You're no longer carrying the weight of the world all alone. You've built a support system; every member brings a unique energy. One that should educate and give you the tools to face challenges head on. An open forum with diverse insight on the best path for your child. It's an invaluable asset. I can't imagine our circle without these MVPs in it.

Till Autism Do Us Part

So often I'm hearing of marriages failing, unable to bear the unrelenting weight that comes when a child is diagnosed. It's understandable. There are so many reasons and often all of them that could be at fault. The shift in priorities, financial strain, guilt, blame, denial.

Those are just the few reasons that took a toll on my marriage—some still do. Aside from the impact to my mental health, I felt tasked with a fundamental responsibility to do right by Jack. I was consumed by all things autism. I read everything about "autism". Research. Data. Forums. Attended any workshop, seminar, support group, or conference offered—some twice. That, coupled with my moral conscious demanding I parent all three of my children in a balanced and just manner, what would be left for us? My husband and I typically are aligned in our parenting styles. We approach most situations as a united front. We strategize before engaging. We rely on each other for support and do our best to divide and conquer with minimal tears shed. Sounds perfect right? As far as parenting, sure, we like to believe we have a handle on that, most days. As a couple? We often fall short. Conflict is certain as hours of sleep decrease, stressors amplify, and behaviours erupt, fracturing any stake we have in unspoken thoughts of *"maybe it's not autism"*. Cracks in the foundation spread like a wildfire.

Patience is a virtue we often could not expend on each other. I found myself sadly preparing for the inevitable despite never envisioning my future with him not in it. We fell into our own routines which rarely included the other. The time we did have together was usually spent laying awake watching the video monitors mounted in Jack's bedroom, anticipating his next curious pursuit. Will he empty every article of clothing onto the floor to leap into like a pile of leaves? Finagle his way around the child proof lid on the coconut oil and lather himself up? Most nights, I watched vigilantly hoping to avoid what typically ends in a 3 a.m. full room sterilization, deep carpet scrub, complete linen change and a "hell hath no fury" style shower for the boy.

Getting out of bed is often the hardest part of my day, and some days I don't. On those days, when I have no more to give, I'm comforted by a gentle embrace and the sweetest words ever spoken, "Stay in bed, Cher. I got the kids". It's those gestures that allow me to recharge for another day and appreciate the luxury of having each other. I empathize with those that have lost their partner for reasons that were of no fault of their own. I admire those who have no fail-safe, yet persevere and meet every new day head on.

When we are gifted with an uneventful night of sleep or sharing a meal *sitting down* I remind myself that we are one of the *"lucky ones"*. For better or worse. Without him, I would have no one to flip a coin with to determine who's turn it is to handle the next inevitable 'shit' storm! All jokes aside, my husband is and has always been the perfect fit to my irregular disposition. He is my refuge and an ally I am blessed with to have on my side.

Small Victories deserve huge celebrations. In Jack's five years, I can recall every bittersweet moment that left me overwhelmed with sadness, gratitude, and sheer joy all at once. I embrace every emotion for what they individually represent. I am grateful to be a part of this amazingly unscripted journey that keeps me in constant anticipation. To experience the indescribable joy I feel when my sweet Jack's eyes light up revealing I've entered into his world. Sharing rare instances when his eyes meet mine, connecting us, even if for the briefest of moments. It breaks my heart in the best way imaginable.

I distinctly recall the day I knew Jack was unique, it was a picture of him no older than four to five months old that told me so. His eyes were focused directly into the camera's lens, a coveted accomplishment for most parents. Yet all that stuck out was his vacant expression, his lack of presence, as though he was looking right through the camera. In spite of my gut feeling, I was unwary of just how telling that photo would prove to be. The neverending series of painful questions that occupy my thoughts every day. Will I ever hear his voice?

Will he ever call me mama? Will I be able to hug and kiss him without causing distress? Every questionable neurotypical development I had with Jack filled me with regret for all the moments I let escape me with my two daughters. I wish I had recognized them then for what they were; blessings. Some days the challenges and tears seem unending, which is why embracing those fleeting moments of clarity is crucial to make it through the long haul. These days we eagerly welcome any event deserving of a celebration, no matter how trivial.

"It is what it is, but it will become what you make it".

I've succumbed to the fact that whether I like it or not, my life has become a "don't try this at home" episode on a loop. There is no way of knowing what to expect on any given day, even in those rare moments when the stars have all aligned, inviting me to exhale, unsuspecting of any uproar because nothing is more reliable than pizza. Cheese pizza, crusts cut off and in bite size squares just like every other third meal before it. Only this time, dependable pizza has ensued pure pandemonium launching a year long boycott. No use questioning what can't be answered, trusty chicken nuggets it is.

Transformation is endless on this journey. It won't always be welcome, but it will be necessary. I'm still often caught by surprise when I should know better and I will forever be challenged with adapting to life's spontaneous escapades, most of which I am not prepared for. We have only just begun our story and most days make me question getting through the chapter. I am exhausted. Emotionally, mentally, and physically. I feel inadequate and defeated. I am vulnerable, uneasy, and sometimes miss the comfort of our once humdrum and predictable life. Our new story is unceasing and yields endless possibilities. It compels me to stretch beyond my comfort zone. But I am still here.

I have experienced immense growth as a mother, wife, and daughter. This impromptu "choose your own adventure" has prized me with purpose and strength to shoulder any challenge I may face. I've been led down a road less travelled and unavoidably chock-full of unknowns. I am no longer sheltered by predictability or conventional means. Accepting what I have no control over is inescapable. My commitment to my children is the only constant I am left with. I love them and that is unchanging.

Move forward, always forward. Find your purpose. Don't plan too far ahead, centre your energy on right now. Immerse yourself in all that is wonderful about your journey. Find the joy in every success and gain wisdom from every setback. Join in on your child's next stim session and experience the most incredible sense of fulfillment. Laugh often and never take yourself too seriously. Every hardship, tear, laugh, success has its purpose even if unrecognizable in the moment. Permit yourself the same consideration you would bestow on another, compassion, patience, understanding and tolerance. One day at a time. There is no pamphlet for the adventure you are embarking on.

For my two beautiful girls, Grace and Sophia. Your unwavering love and devotion for your brother is a direct reflection of the remarkable girls you are and extraordinary women you will become. I am so proud of you both.

Love, Mom

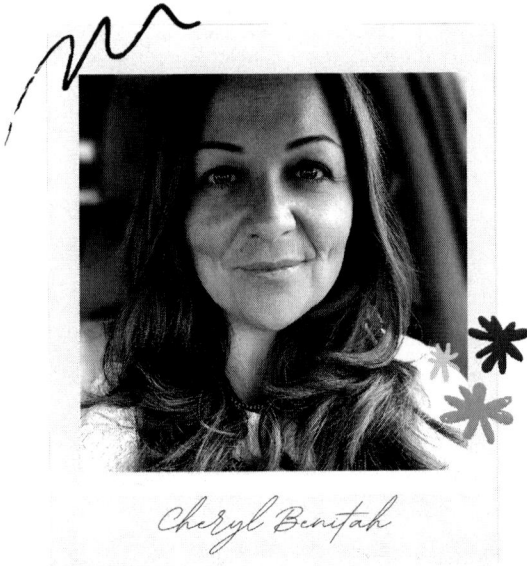

Cheryl Benitah

Cheryl is a 43-year-old mother of three children, one of whom is on the spectrum. Growing up, Cheryl's tenacious personality was both a gift and a curse that often landed her on the heels of mischief. Cheryl's inclination to react impulsively was often viewed as unruly and rebellious. Her adolescent years proved to be charged with self discovery and the compulsion to discredit those who bet against her was the catalyst that inspired her to become a child and youth counsellor. She has dedicated her career to advocate and serve youth with a multitude of struggles. With over 20 years in the field, she has extensive experience in the areas of dual diagnosis, mental health disorders, incarcerated youth, and several years earning her stripes working with high risk adolescents in both hospital and residential settings.

Love Has No Words

By Tara Bourgeois

I grew up in a family of four. My mom and dad, my sister and I. My sister and I are fraternal twins. We are like night and day. She has blonde hair and I have dark brown hair. She was taller than me and was more outgoing, and I was very shy. We had a typical loving family growing up. I met my husband when I was 19-years-old, but we were longtime friends until my late twenties when we became an item. I had my daughter, Carly, at 34 years of age. I had such an easy pregnancy with her and had so much energy. She was a beautiful baby but delivering her was scary. I was rushed into surgery during labor as I spiked a fever of 104 degrees. Turned out I had an in utero infection, so they had to keep my daughter in hospital for five days after delivery to give her the necessary medication.

About four months later I was pregnant again, but unfortunately, into my eighth week I miscarried and lost the baby. Then I got pregnant with my son, Justin, at 36-years-old. My pregnancy with him was very different from my pregnancy with my daughter. He was in a breech position, laying across my stomach. I had constant pains in my sides when I walked too much. Then further along, I became very lethargic. Despite all that, it was all worth it when I first laid eyes on him. He was a beautiful baby.

When my son was about 14-months-old, I started to notice things that were different from my daughter. He never made a noise other than to cry when he was hungry. He stared at our ceiling fan every time we walked by it with him in our arms. He started lining toys up in a row, and he never seemed to acknowledge other kids around him and only played by himself. He also didn't respond to his name or make eye contact. The biggest red flag of all was when he sat there and started moving his arm over and over while staring at it. When I went to the doctor for his checkup, the doctor and I realized he wasn't meeting his milestones for his age, so she sent me to CAMH (Centre of Addiction and Mental Health) to be tested.

While waiting for this appointment, I did countless research to determine what was wrong with my son. As a mother, you want answers so that you can do whatever is necessary to help your child. While researching many of his behaviors, the word "autism" kept coming up. To be honest, it took my breath away and scared me all at the same time. What would I do if it was autism? Could I handle it? What would this mean for his future? Or, for ours as a family? After four months of these agonizing questions, we finally saw the

63

doctor at CAMH. After intensive questions about his behaviors and milestones, the doctor left the room. While we waited I kept telling myself, "I can do this. He's my son and no matter what that doctor comes back to tell me, it won't matter." I just have to look into those beautiful innocent eyes and my heart melts.

As the doctor re-entered the room and took a seat, I took a deep breath and he said, "He doesn't have autism. He scored close to the range but didn't fall into the category." I thought to myself, "What? How can this be? All my research pointed in this direction, and yet it's not autism. If it isn't, what is it then?" He said that he believed that he may have a learning disability. I didn't know what to think or believe from that appointment. I was afraid to say anything since he was a professional, but I felt he was very wrong. My husband agreed with the doctor. Maybe it's my mother's intuition, but I couldn't get it out of my head.

A year passed and we still didn't have any answers to those questions. But then, at one of my son's checkups, our doctor questioned the other doctor's claim that it was not autism. So, she referred me to a developmental pediatrician. He was now three-years-old, and I was extremely nervous about the outcome of this meeting. Once there, she asked me, "What are your concerns with your son?" And so, it began, "I think my son has autism" and then I went on to mention all the behaviors he exhibits. She said to me, "you missed your calling because you are right." She went on to praise me for the lengths in which I went to in order to figure out what was going on with him and stated that not all parents do the research. They just wait until they see the doctor. But for me, I still felt sad though that it took this long to get that official diagnosis.

On my way home, I cried uncontrollably due to the fact that it took this long to get these answers and the real impact of the word "autism" hit me. The bigger questions started to flood in. Not knowing what this would mean for his future. What will happen to him after I'm gone?

Now, the real work began. I was given a world of information at my hands and became overwhelmed. During all this, my husband and I broke up. I think it was too much for him. Someone not worth mentioning said to me once, "You're the reason your son is like this?" Those words stuck with me for a long time and I still think about it at times. A part of me wonders, "Is it something I did while pregnant with him? Did I eat something I shouldn't have?" I found myself trying to recall my whole time pregnant with him to see if there was truth to this. Sometimes I wonder if his autism is from me. I'm an introvert and have trouble with social situations. I don't like being places where it's extremely loud. I was an extremely picky eater as a child. Maybe there's some link there.

Alas, still no answers. Nobody seems to know the answer to that question. It's funny, I think back to my childhood and I don't recall ever hearing the word "autism". Now it's so well known and heard of. When I meet new people, most of them have someone in their family that has autism. I never thought this would be my life. I'm the first one in my family to have a child with autism. I wish we had the answers as to why. I think about it all the time. I wonder if I'll ever know in my lifetime.

So with all this information, where do I begin? Thankfully, Community Living stepped in and helped with filling out countless forms. It was all so overwhelming and I was still trying to get used to this diagnosis that was finally given to my son. Erinoakkids also contacted me and we then started ABA therapy for him through a private centre. But before he started, I had to do a fundraiser because there was no way I could afford to pay for this therapy. I was a stay-at-home mom and since divorced was only receiving spousal and child support. My mom and dad were amazing. They did most of the leg work and got most of the donations. It still brings tears to my eyes when I think about it. They've been my biggest supporters. We managed to raise just over $5,000. So, I started him with two-and-half-hours a day, twice a week, hoping to stretch the money as long as I could. It's a good thing I did because when the money was almost drained dry, the government stepped in and started funding for kids with autism. With the government stepping in, I was able to increase his hours to four-and-a-half-hours, five days a week. This was far better as I soon started to see progress through his learning.

Age four was the time he started school. I won't lie, I had a lot of anxiety leading up to this moment. The reason being was that he is nonverbal and can't tell me if something happens. I didn't have too much anxiety when he started therapy because I felt confident that they could handle him due to their education in this area with autism. I had also heard horror stories from parents about their experiences through the school system which weren't good. But soon my anxiety became less and less as time went by, and I became more confident when in communication with the school.

Since my son was nonverbal, he started learning a PEC (Picture Exchange Communication) system when he was three-years-old. But, unfortunately, by the time he reached age six, he still didn't seem to make any progress in learning. So, my therapist suggested we try him with an iPad using an app called proloquo2go. I thought, "Sure, what do we have to lose?" We weren't getting any progress on the PEC system so it couldn't hurt to try. So, I got an iPad and got everything set up and started to send it to therapy with him each day. They told me since they were going to start teaching him there, it's important that it should be used in all his environments. Okay, I get it.

So, I spoke to the school and told them that we would be starting him with the iPad as the PECs weren't very successful. Well, that didn't go well. They wanted to continue with the PEC system. Well, that infuriated me. How was I going to make this successful when half of his day is spent in school? Then a friend suggested I contact the media. So, I did. Right away, I was contacted by City TV and CTV. Needless to say, by the time it was on TV that day, I received a call and was informed that they would allow him to use it at school. I just couldn't understand why they couldn't allow him to use it at school when this would be his voice. I'm glad I did fight for his right to use it because now at the age of eight-years-old, he has progressed so much with it and now can communicate his needs and wants. Yay! I should add that, unfortunately, during all these struggles, his dad was not there fighting with me. I fought my son's battles alone.

While he was learning to use his iPad, he went through a period of time where he was getting frustrated because of his challenges with communicating those wants and needs. It was a very hard time for me emotionally and physically. My sweet loving boy became very aggressive and abusive. When he wasn't abusing me, he was destroying things around him. At one point, my dad drove two-and-a-half hours from where they live to help me deal with these behaviors. I found myself crying all the time. I went to my doctor and broke down in tears in front of her. She gave me medication to help with my resulting depression. Then she referred me to a doctor for my son, and soon I had him on medication to help.

Eventually, with the new government that was elected, they changed the autism program. So, we had a fight on our hands. Little does the government know, parents of children with disabilities are relentless in fighting and advocating for our children. Yes, I was one of them down on the front lawn of the legislature with my picket sign. In the end, we won a needs-based program and my son received a full day's worth of therapy (seven-and-a-half hours, five days a week). It was a great day. He was around seven-years-old by this time.

The hardest part of my journey with my son and autism is that I always felt alone. No one in my family seemed to understand what I was going through except a select few. I didn't have much support. I didn't have many friends anymore. It isn't easy taking my son out to certain events. Family gatherings, special occasions, birthday parties, and even indoor playgrounds are a struggle for him because he gets upset as soon as we enter the building. A lot of times I stayed home. Many times, I felt like I needed a break, but was never able to have one. Then I voiced my loneliness and despair on an autism group on Facebook and the next thing I know, a wonderful lady invited me to go for coffee. We had so much in common. It was the best day I've had in awhile. She understood my struggles and my tears. Finally, someone who understands and gets my feelings. After that, we started inviting other parents and now there are usually four to six of us. We try to meet once a month. I always look forward to it. I now have a home to go visit through my new found friends that won't make me uncomfortable or judge my son or me.

I feel sorry for my daughter sometimes. She feels like an "only child". I feel bad that I can't always be there in the way she needs me to be because I'm always having to tend to her brother. Every chance I get, I try to make time for her. But sometimes when I get a chance, I just want to rest. I'm exhausted. It's hard being a single parent. My mom says, "God chose you for a reason." That "God only chooses special people for these special children." I want to say, "Then why does it have to be so hard?" But when he cuddles me, or I tickle him and he laughs and then comes back for more, when he's hurt and the only word he ever says is "Mama", those are the moments that make it all worthwhile. If I've learned anything from this journey I'm on, it's that I never knew how strong I was until I was put in this position. Also, that I'm not alone. Many other families are going through the same thing as me. One other thing, I realized I'm more compassionate to others and their struggles. If I see you on Facebook talking about your struggles, I'll reach out, just like someone reached out to me. It's important because we get each other. We all have the same struggles. All this said, I would not change anything. I love my son through the good and bad. He's my life.

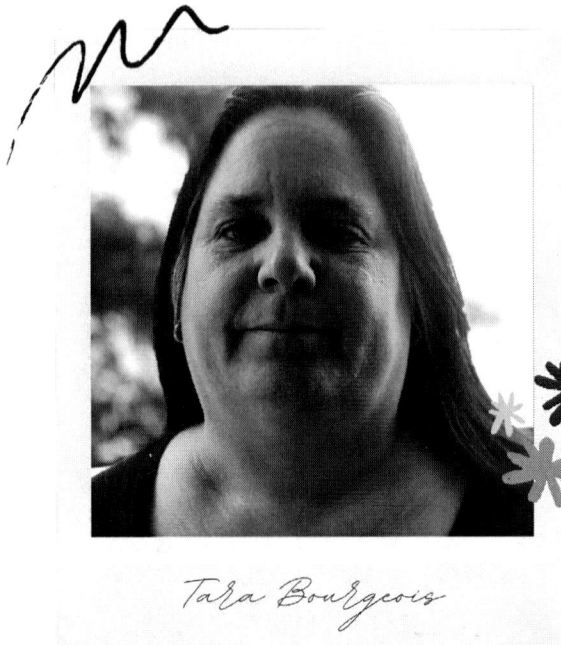

Tara Bourgeois

Born in Toronto, Ontario, Tara completed high school at Thistletown Collegiate Institute in Etobicoke, Ontario and went on to Humber Collegiate institute to complete her secretarial certificate. Tara also became an educational assistant for many years due to her love of children until she became a stay-at-home mom of two children. She's a strong and passionate advocate for autism and is a member of the Ontario Autism Coalition. She loves Canada and its beautiful countryside. She has studied all things related to autism for years upon receiving her son's diagnosis so she could better understand and be a part of his world. "Love has no words" is her strong belief as her son is nonverbal. She is his strongest advocate and will not stop, until her last breath.

Email: tarabourgeois66@gmail.com

The Centre of Us

By Valerie Coates

Adara's Birth

The first time I looked into her eyes was when she was just born into this world. I greeted her with a big smile, her eyes were wide open. As she heard everyone's voices you could see her looking around. She had her Daddy's big blue beautiful eyes and she came zooming into the world saying, "I'm here ready to change your life! Are you ready?" Soon enough, she would really change my entire life. We named that beautiful big blue-eyed girl Adara. Our stay at the hospital was a bit hard as her sugars were a little high, so they had to keep pricking her sweet, little foot, and she would cry out every time. Her sugars did eventually stabilize.

Adara is my second child out of four children. Later on, with my third pregnancy I found out at the time I had gestational diabetes. When the doctor looked back at my pregnancy with Adara, she told me I had borderline gestational diabetes at the time of that pregnancy as well. That information was never disclosed to me from my recollection. Regardless of knowing that, I now have two boys despite the fact that I had gestational diabetes during pregnancy where I controlled it to the best of my ability. Both my boys are healthy and have no conditions at all. And from what we knew as we left the hospital the next day with Adara, we had a healthy, beautiful baby girl.

Baby to Toddler — The Shift

During the infant years with Adara, she was amazing. She slept really well, didn't cry much at all, ate really well, enjoyed fruits, vegetables, and pretty much any food we put in front of her. From infant to toddler years she stood up, walked, ran, waved, used babbling "mamama" and "dadada", to the point of a few words starting to form. The words "bye" and our cat's name, Ruby, by the time she was a toddler. I really can't pinpoint the exact moment where Adara had begun changing. Looking back, I had a lack of complete awareness of where everything changed developmentally. It was sudden and drastic for us. It was all just before the age of two when the way Adara began communicating with us was completely opposite of how things were initially progressing. It started in small ways. Carrying a shovel with her at all times, which was a bit odd. Standing on her tippy-toes and banging her head.

At this time, family members would try and alert me of the signs of autism. I would just respond that she would "get over this" and it was "just a phase". With an ECE (early childhood educator) background, I thought I knew what was best and didn't want to accept others' ideas of what was really happening to our daughter.

Then, it continued: screaming for her sippy cup, chewing on her velcro shoe straps, to the point she would follow me around the house screaming and crying constantly, chewing entire books to shreds. She was no longer interested in eating fruits and vegetables. Her favorite food was crackers and cereal—anything crunchy. Basically, junk and processed foods. I didn't know how to stop what was happening to our sweet baby girl we had brought home that day from the hospital. Who had she become? I was in complete and utter denial and not accepting all these ways in which she was responding to her environment around her.

Denial is one of the stages I learned as an ECE that parents experience. I couldn't see it for myself at the time. I was completely in denial that our beautiful blue-eyed girl had autism. At this point, my sister came to my home and handed me a print out that she researched for where to look for help. I made the call that very day to journey my way to a diagnosis.

Autism Diagnosis—Why Us?

Once we made the call, they directed us to the PEP Start Clinic (Prevention Early Identification Program) which was available in our community. Our top two concerns were that she was not communicating with us and chewing everything. They identified that Adara needed a developmental assessment, had delays in expressive language, receptive language, social communication, play skills, and that there were sensory concerns. This isn't something any parent wants to hear, but the truth was now out and it allowed us to move forward instead of feeling so stuck and unaware of what was happening to Adara.

Now, looking back, I truly feel grateful for finding PEP Start as it helped us get on the pathway of supporting her much earlier, as opposed to waiting an entire year before any developmental assessment would have been done, and six months longer to wait to see the developmental pediatrician to find out if she had autism or any delays. Right after this happened, I made the call to Erin Oak Kids and put our daughter on the waitlist. With that early referral to the organization, we were able help get support with the therapeutic treatment she needed much sooner.

Six months later, the date had arrived and we finally had our appointment with the developmental pediatrician. By this point, the worst of the behaviours had begun: holding in her bowel movements, and shortly after, her "stimming" began. It started out very mild but intensified. When she stimmed, she would freeze. Her hands would raise in the air and she would shake as if having a convulsion, and then run back and forth, over and over again. Depending on the day it could be very frequent—up to 10 or more times a day. To top everything off, she had lost all her verbal development. Her language skills were gone and she was no longer speaking. Everything was screaming and temper tantrums. The stress of this was nothing I had ever experienced before. We had explained all of this to the doctor and left that appointment with a list of all the places to call—which thanks to the PEP Start, some calls were already made—and a recommended stool softener to help with her bowel movements. This didn't help Adara's sensory issue with bowel movements. And lastly, confirmation that yes, our daughter definitely has autism. We received our diagnosis letter two months later which read ASD: autistic spectrum disorder/speech/social/cognitive delay.

One month later, again thanks to the PEP Start Clinic Referral, we were already in getting Adara's speech developmental assessment with Erin Oak Kids, which is our local therapeutic treatment facility for children with developmental disabilities. By this point, Adara is only a couple months away from her third birthday. Can you imagine? Not even three-years-old. A sweet, innocent little girl, and she already has all of these complications? There were many times back then, and sometimes still, I wondered: why us? In the assessment report they wrote "Adara is a sweet 2-year-11-month-old girl who presented with severe delays in receptive and expressive language skills, as well as delays in social communication and play skills." This was really a hard blow, but her Daddy and I were determined for her to get the most support possible.

We went away from Erin Oaks that day confirming the delays that PEP Start identified for Adara, not to mention it was now recognized that she had low eye contact. They also gave us information on recommended workshops that would help us understand what the diagnosis means and ways we could help with all of Adara's behaviours. I found all of the workshops very helpful and we could implement some things into our home to help with her understanding of her environment and how to better communicate with one another. They had many workshops: how to use reinforcement, toileting strategies, understanding behavior, how to use picture exchange communication (PEC), sensory processing, school transitioning. I did them all. Anything that could help her have a better and happier life.

One moment during a workshop that really changed my life was when a parent asked, "What about the child's diet?" And the person in the presentation obviously couldn't answer that. That one question stuck with me. I remember when doing my ECE (Early Childhood Education) the classroom teacher was talking about autism and how families have tried everything to treat autism through diet. Some families even travelled the world for remedies to help cure it. Some even have children who have grown out of it. While I was doing all of these workshops, Adara had started speech therapy with Erin Oaks, so every time there was an opportunity to learn and also consult with the therapists, so I fully engaged in the process. After that workshop she had her speech therapy session and during that I asked the therapist about diet. I will be forever grateful for her answer. She didn't say no! She just said, "Do your research!"

Research, Research, Research!

Disclaimer: I am not a doctor, I do not treat, diagnose or suggest any of these next things you will read. I made a decision to go down this rabbit hole so that I could make the best choices and decisions for my child's disability. Proceed with an open mind and if you want to know more, it's best to consult with a professional in this area of expertise.

And research is what I did! Every night, once all the kiddies were in bed, my laptop would be on my lap and I read and read and read. People's testimonials as to how they have helped their child just by diet change and supplementations. On YouTube, I watched many videos that talked about autism recovery. I did a lot of reading about DAN (Defeat Autism Now) doctors, biomedical treatment, clean diet, leaky gut, heavy metal toxicity, and vaccinations.

I chose to start making changes to our diet. Our clean diet included being yeast-free, no artificial sugar, gluten, and dairy/casein free. Initially, I started a gluten-free diet and started shopping only on the outskirts of the grocery store in the natural food sections for my family based on my research on how to make the gluten-free shift and go more towards whole foods. After we had weaned all of the wheat-based foods out of our home and started incorporating more whole foods, we slowly started to notice a shift in Adara's awareness.

At this time, she was in preschool to help her socially. I would personally prompt her when she should say "hi" and "bye" and we had incorporated music therapy once per week for just 30 minutes per session. During music therapy sessions she responded extremely well, and for the most part, with redirection, she loved to engage with the instruments. About three months after being gluten-free, Adara was now saying "Hi" and "Bye", as well using some sign language. This led us to finally finding an integrative doctor that had a DAN certification. Now, this isn't to say that I want my daughter to not be autistic, as I have grown over the years. And this isn't about her "getting over it". I just wanted her to be okay and be able to function as best as she could for her and her life. DAN certified doctors use the practice of biomedical treatment for people who are diagnosed with ASD.

Biomedical treatment is treating the body in some of the following ways: supplementation, special testing, detoxification, and dietary changes. A great place to get lots of information is the Healing Hope Tribe. They post many videos on YouTube where they talk in depth about biomedical treatment.

Leaky gut and yeast overgrowth are things that appear in many children with autism which are said to affect or intensify symptoms. Leaky gut happens when the yeast affects the inner walls of the digestive system to the point that different pathogens can leak through the walls and get into the bloodstream, affecting vital organ parts. Adara did have this and it showed through her bowel movements (BM).

To begin with, she had major sensory issues with her BMs, and it did get to a point that when she did have a BM it would be very inconsistent, watery, and sandy. Food was not totally broken down. Now, I understand that her body wasn't digesting the food properly. One of the ways that we treated that was through simply using probiotics that the integrative doctor recommended. Months later, her BMs were at a regular consistency, and by the time she was six-years-old, she was fully toileted. I highly recommend looking into the behavioural signs of leaky gut as they are so diverse and seemingly unrelated that you might not make the connection to the real issue. Symptoms such as headaches, sleep disturbances, hyperactivity, and even toileting resistance can all potentially be related back to leaky gut.

Heavy metal toxicity is a buildup due to the environment that is around the child. We can become exposed to heavy metals from many different sources such as air, water, foods, medicines, and from industrial pollution. Adara had heightened lead levels. Thankfully, it wasn't in the red zone but very close to it.

Again, I recommend digging deeper into heavy metals as they can cause a large variety of symptoms such as headaches, vomiting, and even neurological problems such as seizures. It is not something to take lightly.

Since then, Adara has had hair testing which read that all her heavy metals are now within a normal range. I can associate a few things on that list that were apparent in her such as pale skin, anemia (low iron), behaviour problems, and school performance. And though, it may be hard to read things like this as a mom, when making decisions I am now more educated and aware. It really has helped me to once again make the right wellness decisions for her.

Vaccinations are a touchy subject and very controversial to say the least. I'm not going to throw out any names or suggest much of anything, but for me it became a very conscious decision that we felt best for our child.

From 2010 to 2012 my daughter was vaccinated eight individual times, under the age of two. There is really something wrong with that in my opinion. As a parent, society tries to tell us it's the right way, the right thing to be doing, and we simply need to follow what they tell us. Now, I choose not to vaccinate and make the choices that I feel are right for my kid's health and wellbeing. I encourage research to be done in regards to this subject as it is a very important topic that every parent should be well-versed in prior to making any decision for their child. Once I did my research, my own personal choice and conscious reasoning was to no longer vaccinate my children.

All of the learnings and research has helped us see where imbalances lie and how to then balance that out. I now know and believe this as well from seeing how Adara has changed over the years just by simply changing her diet, giving supplements, and using specialized testing. It really led me to understand that what happened to her was that her body became burdened, could no longer detoxify itself and the many toxins which built up over time, and caused a neurological problem in our child. The brain is the control centre to how we behave and respond to the world. But if a brain is being attacked by all of these toxins in the body, it breaks down. It becomes damaged. We are after all organic as well, and just like a plant. If it's not watered or given healthy soil, it can become unwell. All of the research, as well as seeing Adara change immensely, pointed to her body being malnourished and overburdened by the environment around her. There is power in finding the truth.

After all of this, Adara was yet again diagnosed. This time it was with epilepsy disorder in 2017. This brought a whole new awareness into our lives as now we had to learn about epilepsy and be aware of what is causing this in her.

Some of the things that we noticed triggers her stress, chemicals—whether it was something sprayed or put on her body like nail polish—and artificial sugar or whatever had been put in the candy such as dyes.

Through this secondary diagnosis, it has led us to now encompass a chemical-free lifestyle to ensure that her brain health is supported, not just nutritionally, but also by the air that she breathes in. I found great education about all of this through an amazing organization called Young Living which has amazing products that are formulated without the use of harsh chemicals. They are plant-based and mineral-based which allows us to have many products that support her health without triggering seizure-related activity.

This has been an ongoing battle to this day as the medical system only wants to medicate people to treat this and not look at what the underlying problems truly are. This is why I will always be continuing my search, reaching out to specialists, and naturopathic doctors who can support us and ensure the best wellness support for her entire wellbeing. I will always advocate for the full wellbeing of my daughter and my entire family's lives.

Spiritually Blessed!

Going through all of this with my daughter has blessed me with a purpose-driven life to provide a pathway for other families who are looking for answers, information, and resources to support families living with autism. Maybe even just to point those who are needing help in the way of researching and finding the information for themselves and choosing to help their child in a way they feel is right. There is no right or wrong way. Everyone has the right to their opinions and what they see is best for their child and family.

Adara has allowed me to know our children are the centre of us. We choose children to help us and guide us. She has shown me something that I never dreamed of having an awareness and an understanding of. She has made me an advocate and a true believer that we, as a community, have to help one another. She brought out my reason and purpose. She has been my reason and purpose. She helped me to see the truth of who we are and the truth in the world! Our child truly is the center of us. These children are truly important beings that need to be cherished for they are bringing forth our truest selves.

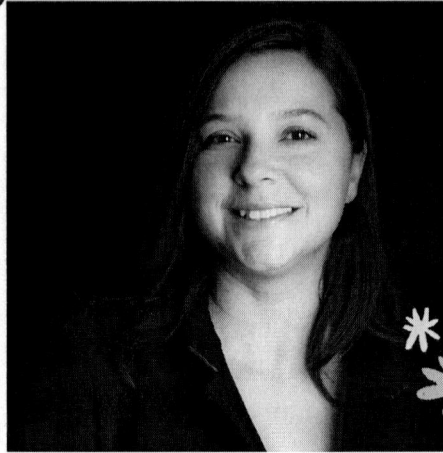

Valerie Coates

Valerie Coates is Owner and Founder of ADARA'S Foundation, a non-profit organization which supports families who have children living with ASD (autism spectrum disorder) and advocates for ASD. Valerie is also a stay-at-home parent to four wonderful children. During the past three years, she has been facilitating Child and Parent Social Groups where families can meet to support their child's aspects of social development while educating families about wellness. ADARA'S Foundation was inspired by her daughter who is diagnosed with ASD. Having gained valuable experience with her daughter has allowed Valerie to consult with families to support them with their child's wellness path. Valerie graduated as an early childhood educator through Sheridan College where she first started to realize her love for working with children. She later did go on to work as an early childhood educator through the YMCA. During her free time, she also passionately focuses on taking care of her family and advocates for living a toxin-free life using Young Living Essential Oils.

Email: adarasfoundation@gmail.com
Facebook: https://www.facebook.com/theautismprocess/

The Ebb and Flow of Life

By Veronica Gaboury

Several years ago at the start of this, when I was feeling overwhelmed and rudderless, what do I wish I would have known then that could have helped me to get to this point now? Would I have listened? While I would have read ideas about advice, I might not have taken it. Especially if the ideas were about what I am going to tell you. That advice is this: you have to take care of you, as the parent, as a care-taker. I am a cautionary tale for what happens if you don't. All I was looking for at the beginning was how to help my daughter and anything else seemed selfish and a waste of time I could be using to help her.

When Kath was first diagnosed, I knew myself well enough to know that what I needed was reading and hearing from other folks who traveled along a similar path, that life would be okay. So, I scoured the Internet and found the blog of a mom who had a daughter with a similar (at the time) diagnosis, and as I read from her past-to-present, I saw a beautiful life unfold. Not a tragic diagnosis taking over someone's life. I also found an online support group, CHASA (Children's Hemiplegia and Stroke Association). And that group, especially its founder, Nancy Atwood, and many of the mothers who have become friends, helped me through some dark and scary times. At one point I even spoke to a few moms with the idea that we would write our own book about Warrior Moms. I felt we were Warriors trying to fight for our children with diagnoses. But, because life got busy, although I never lost my hope to write, other things took up the energy and time. Until I find myself here, 12 years later. Looking back, I can see a kind of road that hopefully I can map for others.

Let's go back to before Kath was diagnosed the first time, perhaps my story mirrors yours. I knew something was "wrong" but I did not have any idea what it could be, and I was oblivious to how big it could be. I was a mom of four children. I was happy, and overwhelmingly busy. I have two sons from my first marriage, and two from my current husband. I always somehow knew that I would have two boys and two girls, so I felt complete. However, that wholeness did not exempt me from feeling completely and utterly in over my head every day with the multiple directions each member of my family was going in.

The boys were bound for college that fall, my husband was ambitious, and then there were the two young girls. Before the girls were born, I had been looking to become more of a leader at my school and taking on more responsibilities as a more senior member of my high school. But once they were born, I decided instead to job-share, which meant I was home every other day with the girls, and I taught on the alternate days. I often felt like I was full time in both places. There was no 'prep' time. My husband did not come home and take over so I could grade, rest, or exercise. I was the one called if the girls were sick. I was on-call 24/7 and the one who made sure the girls had a caretaker when I wasn't able to be home. I was the one trying to understand the ebb and flow of having older children who are beginning to spring out of the nest. I was really in over my head.

As my oldest son, Chris, prepared to study abroad for a semester in Nicaragua, and my other son, Nick, went off to his first year of college, I really began to notice my youngest daughter, Kath, was missing all of her developmental milestones. Not just one or two. All. Kath was happy, she was loved, but she was not moving the way she should have. After Chris and Nick went off to their different paths, at Kath's yearly physical, I brought my concerns up with our pediatrician, Dr. Schottler. And although she said she didn't see anything too off track, she trusted her parents to recognize when something wasn't quite right. She set up an early intervention visit by our county to test Kath immediately. The therapists came to our home a few weeks later and before they left they said she definitely qualified for services, and although they couldn't diagnose her, Kath was displaying obvious delays.

A few weeks later Kath began therapy in our home and we saw some immediate improvements. Then we visited a developmental neurologist who spoke to us, watched Kath, examined her, and sent us off for more testing. We were fortunate that an opening for an MRI opened up that week and we didn't have to wait the agonizing two months for our appointment. The results came back the next day that Kath had survived an in utero stroke. She also presented with having mild right-sided hemiplegia.

One thing that our developmental neurologist told us immediately was, "Don't go on the internet to look this up, wait until we talk on Monday" and the second bit of advice was "Never limit her." To say that I felt untethered with Kath's diagnosis would be just the start of understanding what I was feeling. It was as though my brain imploded. How could this be? How could an unborn baby have a stroke? Yes, I was an older mom at 37, but I did not drink or do drugs. I followed doctors' orders. I ate well. But it did not matter. I had a daughter who was always going to have to struggle with life and it happened while she was inside of me. I blamed myself.

I went online immediately and researched, despite the doctor's warning. Some information was terrifying, as the doctor suggested. But as I mentioned, one mom's blog helped me feel hope and possibilities. This diagnosis was not a death sentence. There were many more health issues involved in this diagnosis as we discovered over time, but I was also old enough to know that even without a diagnosis of this magnitude, it hadn't meant that we would be exempt from anything either. I wish I had saved that mom's blog because I should have told her the impact of her sharing her story had on me—which is one of the most important reasons behind me wanting to write and share something of our journey here, in addition to my own blog. Perhaps I can give someone else some hope.

However, despite the hope that mom handed to me, I struggled. We had two other major health issues going on at the time: my son had an accident two years prior that left him with a traumatic brain injury (TBI), and even when he went off to college, we didn't understand its ripple effects; my husband had a roll-over car accident in a snow storm two weeks after Kath was diagnosed, the month after we paid off his car and had just taken the collision coverage off of his car, and he also had a TBI. We were already struggling with our budget from my part-time position for job sharing, a growing family, and growing obligations, but we began to drown financially, despite a friend giving us a gift to research therapies (a forever thank you to the Collins). We looked into hippotherapy specifically, as well as dance and music. I was struggling with the fact that I could not help anyone.

If people around me saw what I was going through, they didn't say anything, but it was likely because I was really good at hiding my struggles. I was having issues with anxiety, but I tried to hide it. I was researching, looking up all sorts of therapies for Kath, but I stopped taking care of me. I often would say things like, "We have to put the oxygen mask over our own faces first as moms" but I did not follow through myself. Anything that made me look weak, I hid. I pushed it all so far down.

I was stretched out of shape with worry for my family's health issues and financial strain; the only reprieve was sleep, but that was also around the time when my sleep habits deteriorated. I woke up during the night to check on the girls (the boys have their own places). Alex, my eldest daughter, had asthma and was often sick and she caught every germ that passed through each grade, and Kath just made me anxious. Our sump pump had to be turned on manually every couple of hours during certain weather and our wood stove had to be fed every three to four hours. I also woke up when Kath couldn't sleep and I'd sleep on her floor, on a makeshift bed of blankets, holding her until we got a full size bed for her room; Alex often joined us, too. Roger was working a second job and due to the nature of his job, which was driving and delivering papers in the early morning hours, he needed uninterrupted sleep, so he was unable to help.

At school I did my job, then ran home and took care of everything at home. We had up to 13 therapies a week for awhile, which meant that my friend Robin who watched the girls every other day, and I had to work Kath through the transitions of sometimes three therapies in one day, while practicing everything she worked on in the other therapies, and still try to let her and Alex be kids who played and were just kids.

My research led to looking into alternative therapies. I drove once a week to hippotherapy. The stable was an hour and 15 minutes away, Kath worked with the horse for 20-30 minutes, (Alex often had a sibling-lesson) and then we drove the hour and 15 minutes ride home. Since the boys were living their own lives, it was only a matter of balancing all of Kath's therapies, alongside what Alex needed. Alex embraced dance and I made sure she had dance classes. We were again fortunate that as Kath watched her big sister, she too wanted to dance, and Kath has always been embraced as herself at her level at the dance studio, as well.

There was so much that was simply just existing on my end, to ensure a better chance and opportunities for the girls. I got really, really lost and I didn't even notice. I tried to maintain some of my professional goals, but if the girls got sick, or there was a specialist appointment to attend, my priority was to parent.

The boys went through some struggling times as well and I am ashamed and embarrassed to say that I was not there for them. I didn't even recognize when they were struggling at times. They had to deal with several issues that I should have been much more present and aware of, but I was unable to.

I was having memory issues by this point too. I began to struggle with remembering everything, except the basics. I could no longer remember the story I was writing. I would get in the car and forget where I was going and how to get there. I even forgot one time that a mom had asked me to bring her daughter home from the dance studio. I was five minutes away from the studio on my way home before I remembered. The girl was safe, but to this day I still have a tough time going into the studio, I am still so mortified. I forgot to grade papers. I forgot to attend meetings, unless they were for my daughters. I forgot the special days at school, the spirit days, and the days I was supposed to send Alex in with certain themes. I forgot to pay bills. More than once I forgot to pay my insurance. I was not taking care of myself, not exercising, and not eating right nor drinking enough water. I couldn't write, I couldn't read, I didn't have time to meet with friends. I could only afford a sitter to work.

If I look back at pictures from that time period, my house was an absolute mess. Piles everywhere. Too much stuff. Don't get me wrong, it's still a mess, but wow, it was intensely disorganized. I remember apologizing to each therapist who came in the door and they said, "This is nothing, it's obvious you care for and love your children. You should see some houses we go into." And I looked around and saw my piles and my messes and my smiling, laughing, goofy kids and thought, "Okay, one day I'll regain control, for now they and these therapies are what's important."

The thing is that Kath's diagnosis was really a family diagnosis. It impacted everyone. First, because everyone now had a daughter or a sister who we knew was going to face challenging obstacles, and what we did now, therapies and opportunities, during her early years was important for whatever she would be able to accomplish for the future. It impacted Alex because it was at a time when she was also growing and needed a lot of guidance, but I was out of focus and distracted. It impacted the boys because they felt badly they weren't around often to help, and I could not negotiate through anything they were dealing with, be it financial aid, student loans, care packages, or support in any way. It impacted Roger and he retreated into his two jobs as a way to feel he was helping, and I was not a reliable partner as a wife. It was as if my brain had folded in on itself and I could only handle little bites of anything.

I began to feel as though I only had so much energy and strength and I could no longer, not only remember things, but I also did not have the ability to be friends with anyone. Friendship took an effort I could not share or expend. I had one friend from before for a while who did help me through, she also had a child with health issues. But even trying to volunteer at the girls' school, I could only do self-contained projects, basic things that I could actually see and understand what was going on. I could not plan anything, take an officer position in the PTA, or even have the energy to attend meetings. I was a Daisy Leader for a period of time, fully embracing the 12-year commitment, feeling I would get better as time went on and the activities became more important, but because I was unable to do as much as some moms wanted, I was asked to step down. I felt alone and adrift and continued to put on a façade of having my act together and knowing what I was doing, but I was losing confidence.

It must seem like I am exaggerating, but none of our family lives close by, so no one saw that I was struggling. Friends will only send you so many invites before they stop. I did participate in a writing project and felt full lungs of air and possible creativity expand in my folded-in brain, but as soon as the three-week workshop ended, the daily reality was that I was needed to be home for the big and the little moments and creativity takes time to work on, and there was no time for that luxury.

As time has continued, as it always does, things have shifted and changed. Things have progressed, lots of aspects of our daily life have improved. We have had a change in diagnosis, developmental growths have altered many routines, and I have learned a lot and we have a lot of joy and happiness.

As time has gone on, the boys have moved on with their lives. I still feel I missed out greatly on some of their most integral parts of being and I can never ever make that up to them, but I do hope they can one day understand that I truly was doing the best I could with what I had at the time. They have moved on to becoming wonderful, empathetic humans who know the value of human connections.

As time has gone on, Alex learned how to work around me, she learned she needed to keep track of her own activities, dates, homework, projects, meetings, and that she often needed to remind me of anything important. I often kidded that we were born in the wrong order, that she should have been the mom. We worked together on having a calendar book and a calendar in the kitchen. She knows that even now I can't remember everything, so she reminds me. I apologize often and she shrugs and tells me it is okay. She is a beautiful old soul. She accepted me as I was, and still does, even as she maneuvers through high school.

As I slowly started to get back to being myself (it has been a slow slough through, but I do feel my memory improving with sleep and more self-care), she is slowly letting go of having to take care of so much. She is still one of the most responsible humans I know, but I do feel bad for forcing her to have to grow up so fast and needing to do so in that way. I believe her anxiety is from all that was laid on her, but we are working on that as well. She is an academic, an artist, a writer, a dancer, and the best big sister Kath could have. She is one of the most empathetic humans who wants to make the world a more accepting place.

As time has gone on, my husband and I have weaved through this like two people dancing to different music and doing different dances. We have struggled with how one another handles the stress; we have grown separately, and we have lost the core of who we are as a couple. We have forgotten how to talk to one another, how to handle one another, how to laugh with one another, and how to parent together. But especially how to be decision-makers and partners together.

We have basically lived parallel lives for the last 12 years. There were long stretches of time where we didn't even sleep in the same bed because someone had to stay near Kath and he needed the sleep so he could work the second job. But we have stayed together when we might have found it easier to leave. Sometimes I think if it wasn't for our financial situation, we would have left one another, but we were too broke, we both love our home, and we are too stubborn. We stayed also because every now and again we would see glimpses in one another of what made us take that initial step to join our lives, it would flicker and although undoubtedly, one of us would blow it out instead of fanning it, we saw it and we both stayed. It is still a challenging dance, but there is also a peace and a grace that comes from knowing that as much as we push and pull one another, neither of us gives up on the other. When we have our moments of clarity, we still do actually choose one another after all.

As time has gone on, Kath has learned to persevere through academic struggles (although the eight times table was purgatory, she could not get the hang of it), physical challenges (a leg brace, hunched over posture, tiredness), social challenges (her voice sometimes is high pitched and her big laugh are 'tells' that can often separate her from peer friendships). And then at the end of fifth grade and half-way through sixth (first year in middle school) she began having other health issues. She was having blurry vision episodes that we thought were optical migraines. She was also having what we thought were night terrors where she woke and didn't know what was going on and didn't remember the next morning, but was flailing and yelling, "No!"

Finally, after months of not knowing what was going on, not having a set diagnosis, Kath spent three days in the hospital, and 11 years after her original diagnosis, she had an extended video EEG, and had her more recent MRI re-read, and it was discovered she has epilepsy and optical migraines. They also found her original diagnosis of having survived a stroke was incorrect, she didn't have a stroke, but rather she has two brain malformations: polymicrogyria and cerebral heterotopia. Thanks to improvements in technology we have many new facets of Kath's brain to study and understand. Thanks to new technology and research there are more options for therapies. But Kath is much more than her diagnosis, her smile lights up a room, her laugh is infectious. She works so hard to learn each new concept or skill. She looks for the good in everyone. She loves to read, play with the dogs, and run. She makes the world a better place.

The past year we have been dealing with learning about the new diagnoses, but the thing is, the world doesn't stop. Even though you are breathless and bruised, it keeps going. Sometimes I come down really hard on myself. Why can't I have the energy of others? Stay as organized as others? Being diagnosed this year with Hashimoto's disease and finding that my thyroid has been fighting against me, has taught me that I need to really take care of myself. No lip service. I researched for myself and I have worked hard at improving: my sleep, my food choices, my hydration, and even exercising, or at least moving my body more. I am not anywhere where I should be, but I have felt a big improvement in my ability to handle stress, in my brain fog and memory, and in my relationships.

What do I want someone to know who is going through a challenging time? I'm still learning, so who am I to give advice? I feel as though I still struggle the most with being so out of control of everything. My bills get out of hand, sometimes we weave into very troubling times with finances. My school work piles high. House stuff is messy. I no longer believe I could handle a position of authority or control, like being a curriculum leader or more, at this point, because I could never make it a priority for my time, energy, and my brain. I try to write and then I forget. That meme about having so many tabs open and not knowing where the music is coming from? That's me. I have lists, then I get sidetracked by more lists, and then I remember the original list, and I am lost.

I don't know, what could I tell someone who is going through a diagnosis? What could I, with all of this chaos in my wake, advise someone about how to handle it all? Maybe this: it could help you to hear from someone in the weeds like me that nothing is completely ever in control. Absolutely nothing. People know that to a certain extent, but when you have a child with a disability, or a diagnosis, it becomes even more obvious. So you might clench the other parts of your life and try to wrangle them into submission, but then that part pops out-of-control, and like a leak in a hose, you notice new spots leaking. Nothing is ever completely in control and eventually you realize, that's okay.

I would also suggest grace. Give yourself grace. I am not religious so I mean more of the kind of grace to forgive yourself when you lose it or when you mess up. Grace when others lose it and make a mistake. Grace for it all. And mean it.

Also, when a branch is thrust in your peripheral as you are being dragged downstream, reach out and grab on. I was always afraid to admit or show I couldn't handle it all. One day at school, the teacher across the hall gave me a card. I don't recall what it said or what it was for, but it was a card that showed me I was seen in my struggle. I normally would smile and say thanks as I was yanked towards the waterfall, but for some reason beyond what I understand about myself, I did reach out that time. And this colleague's friendship has continued to sustain me. Thanks, Jeff. And thanks to the other very special parts of my new inner circle, namely Mary, Caroline, Cathy, Kristine and Colleen, Cara, Christine, and Darlene, who have never been frightened away, who check on me, and also give me branches to hold on.

In line with the previous thought, I suggest you ask for help when you need it. Talk to someone, write a journal, have someplace to turn to when you are overwhelmed. And it's okay to need help, whether it's help picking the kids up from school, help filling out a form, taking care of the bills, or stopping the world for a few minutes to grab a cup of coffee. You would help anyone else who needed it, right?

Another piece of advice, stop blaming yourself. Stop blaming anyone else. What you have is energy to help your child, you don't have energy to spare on such draining energies. We have no idea why Kath was born with her issues. I don't always take my advice, I do often still blame myself, and the environment, and the negative thoughts I might have had during the pregnancy. But my daughter, my family, needs me right now, right here, and that negative blaming-kind of thinking takes away from any positive energy and actions I may be able to do.

I wish I knew it was a marathon that would always feel like it was at a sprint pace. I wish I had known that I would never 'catch-up' that I would always have something slightly out of reach, some green light on the dock across the Sound, Gatsby-like. I wish I knew that some folks who I thought would never turn away, would. And as painful as that was, it was alright to try to fix it, then to grieve it, and then to move on. I wish I could hug that Veronica, who stood in the dining room listening through the phone about Kath's initial diagnosis. I wish I could hug her and say, "Pace yourself. Forgive the times you will flounder as quickly as you would forgive others. Embrace and enjoy the moments in between the panic gasps, they are the air in your lungs. Work harder at friendships, you will need them. Take care of yourself, it's not selfish, it's survival. You might not always be as prepared as you like, but that's okay. You will be happy in your new normal. Your family needs you, more than they need the house clean, or things in control. You got this. You got this, even when you don't, you got this." You got this, too.

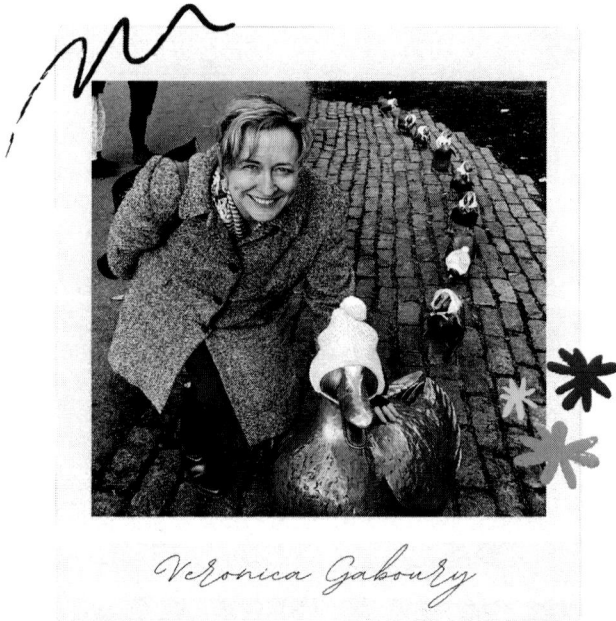

Veronica Gaboury

Veronica Steiger-Gaboury has been a mom for over 30 years, and a writer for even longer. Although each of her four children have presented her with a variety of life adventures, her youngest daughter has taught her a different lens to see the world and Life's Adventures through. As a high school teacher and a mom, Veronica often blogs and posts on social media about the sometimes rollercoaster paths having a child with different learning abilities and strengths, as well as health issues, can do to one's family, and one's sense of self, as she tries to make sure that her daughter gets everything she needs to reach her own best self.

You can read more about our journey on my blog, "Attempts at Clarity" http://vsstuff.blogspot.com/

Everyone Has a Talent

By Danella Hesler

My Story

Here is just a part of my story. Two weeks before I was born, my mother fell down three flights of stairs. The stairs hit either my head or my mother's head. When I was born the "experts" told my parents that I would have difficulty with math, reading, and writing. Their most optimistic prediction was that I might make it to Grade 8. School was the one place I never wanted to be—I was bullied almost every day, especially after my best and only friend moved away. I discovered that I could make myself sick with respiratory infections just to get out of going to school.

As a young child, I once heard a minister say that everyone had a talent, and it was a gift. He said we needed to use that gift to the maximum for the good of all. Wow! What about me? If I had a talent, what was it? I began to read books on history, geography, and people that did amazing deeds.

Going to high school just seemed like a long road, full of more problems and I decided to go to a private school. I had friends there and no bullies. In Grade 12, we had to do the SATs (Scholastic Aptitude Test) however, I said I was planning on being a garbage man or a plumber so I would not need to do that test. The principal, unfortunately, disagreed and said I had to do it. Sometime later that year in the middle of English class, the principal interrupted the class to announce that I had fooled him for the last time. He informed everyone that I was in the top 4% of all students that completed the SAT test. I was astounded to say the least. He, on the other hand, was very upset because he had believed, as had I, that I could barely learn. Strangely though, I could read books that others never would read; all the books by L.M. Montgomery, Leo Tolstoy, Dostoevsky, Victor Hugo. I read anything that spoke of the plight of humanity.

Learning this new information that I had some intelligence now had me more perplexed. The more I pondered on my abilities the less I could figure out what I really wanted to do. Eventually, I chose chef training and I obtained a job after graduation. Over the years I had many types of jobs from cooking demonstrator, to instructor of mentally challenged adults, to owning a bakery. I got married and had two children.

Still, the search to know more was deep in me. Then, one day, an accident happened to me at work. A wall fell on my head. It was a glass block wall that measured 3 feet by 5 feet high. Now, suddenly I was in pain all the time. I could not turn my neck and my back was so tight even breathing was a problem. One day I found a flyer for Mitzvah and I decided to go the next day. I began to regain flexibility, and the pain was going away. The Mitzvah teacher I went to told me I needed to learn this work. I thought to myself that there was no way I could sit still and memorize body "stuff". But I soon discovered this was different. This was hands-on learning. The instructor demonstrates by moving your arms or legs and then you take a turn to try it on them.

That was my way to learn—a real hands-on experience. I took the course for three years and graduated, and that started me on a path to constantly learning unusual information about our bodies.

Alternative Ideas for Well-Being

In this section, I would like to give people some alternative ideas that they may not have heard about. This is not just for the child, but as well for all the parents that I have ever met who are stressed to the max. Just letting go of tension in their body can change the stress dynamics in the family.

Body Movement

There are many types of movement and energy healing modalities. These are the ones which I am most familiar with. I never see these mentioned in books or articles, so it may give you new choices for contributions to you and your child's well being.

Reiki

Reiki has several levels of classes and there are Reiki masters. It is an energy around the body and it is not necessary to touch the person. Some teachers do put hands on specific areas, and some do not.

Mitzvah Technique

Mitzvah Technique was created by my teacher, Nehemiah Cohen. He first learned "Alexander work" and over time he developed Mitzvah. In this work it means a gift to the giver. As a Mitzvah teacher you receive what you have given to someone else's body. There are two parts of Mitzvah. One is movement exercises and the other is hands-on body work. Both are gentle, slow movements allowing the body to release deep-set tension and stress. Flexibility and mobility increase with this work. The body work is done on a massage table with the person fully clothed. Mitzvah teachers are mainly in Canada and Japan. There is a three-year certification course required to become a Mitzvah practitioner.

All the children I worked with between the ages 8 to 23 loved body work and because my specialty is the Mitzvah Technique, that was what they received in my office. Although hugging was not their thing, and it is not mine, the love of having their body moved would bring out statements like, "Why are you finished?" and "When am I coming back?" and "Can I live with you?". One boy that came to my office the first time stood outside the door for the first 15 minutes. Then, when he did enter the office he never wanted to leave.

Access Consciousness Bars

Using gentle touch on 32 specific spots on the head that allows an electric discharge to occur and new neural connections to be created. It is a set of tools that are designed to facilitate more change for everyone. This work was created by Gary Douglas.

Other types of modalities

Radionics

For a nine minute video of the machines I use check out my website at www.mitzvah.ca or by searching YouTube for "radionics". It is a method of using photons of light and sound waves to find any type of inflammation in the body and it will destroy what is creating that inflammation. This work uses a sample of hair to identify the invader/problem as well as send a session. The person does not have to be present in the room for this session. The hair is connected to the machine which has multiple dials to identify body organs and systems, as well as the cause of the problem. The machines utilize numeric codes that have taken over 60 years of research to identify and calibrate. Each machine has 108 dials and the radionics practitioner will use the codes in specific sequence to transmit the photons to the person wherever they may be.

My daughter Milica and I have several types of radionics machines. Some with Scalar waves and other types that are more for bone and joint problems.

Homeopathy

A homeopathic person takes many years of education to understand personalities and which remedy works for specific types of people. It is not the "disease" but rather the pattern of the individual that makes the remedy choice. There are homeopathic practitioners in every state and province in the US and Canada.

Please note, I have personally used these modalities for my own health and well being.

Our Children Are Amazing Beings

I still get stressed by writing. This is one of the most stressful things I could do. But when Rose-Anne asked me if I would think about contributing my story, I hoped it would let anyone that read this know there are choices that we do not always know about. I am constantly learning about new methods and ideas. And to also look at our children and know they are amazing beings full of possibilities that are waiting to be discovered.

The point I am making is you never know what you or your child showed up to create on this planet and what contribution you and your child can be for others.

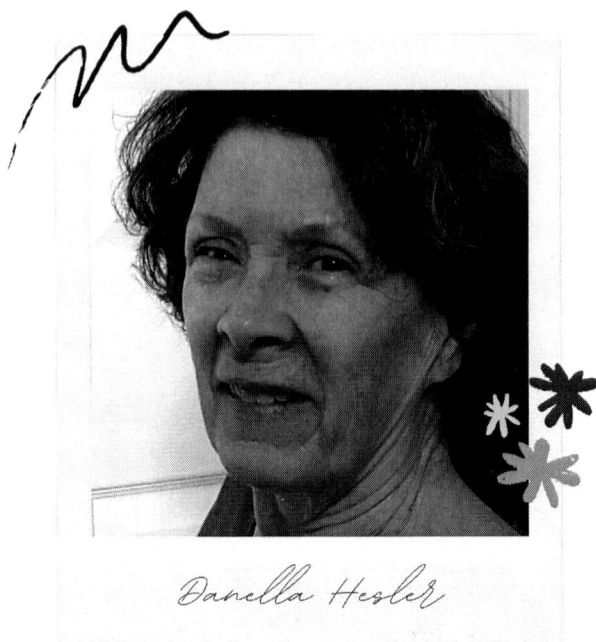

Danella Hesler

When Danella was born, her parents were told her ability to learn would be limited and she would probably not be able to do math or write. They predicted she would have speech problems and someone would have to look after her all her life. They were wrong. Later, Danella was a 38-year-old chef in pain when she went for a Mitzvah Technique session in Toronto. That day was the beginning of life without pain. Her sciatic pain of 17 years was gone. In addition, Danella's curiosity turned to radionics. Funded through a non-profit group, Danella helped 15 children with learning disabilities receive weekly radionics sessions over two years and they had many improvements over that time. In 2007, Danella received a Doctorate of Natural Medicine.

To contact Danella:

Email: danellahesler@aol.com
Website: www.mitzvah.ca

You Are Braver Than You Believe

By Diana Mostoway

> *"You are braver than you believe, stronger than you seem, and smarter than you think"*– movie *"Pooh's Grand Adventure: The Search for Christopher Robin" (1997),* written by *Karl Geurs and Carter Crocker*

My story as Caroline's mom, as someone who discovered and now raises a child who has autism, is a story about me as much as it is about her—my character, my marriage, my role as a parent. Everything was challenged, and many things were challenging. All I know is that I can do it. And so can you if you are in a similar situation. I won't say that everything will work out fine–but I will say, you can do it. If you do, there is much hope for you and your child. I overcame so much, and I ended up believing in myself as much as I believe in my daughter Caroline. If you have newly discovered that you have a child with special needs, then you need to know that I believe in you, too.

In the Beginning

I tried to have a baby for years. Caroline was born in July, in the middle of the night, our long-awaited miracle. She seemed so peaceful that first night I could hardly see if she was breathing. Of course, I poked her, woke her up, just to be sure. I had all the possibilities in front of me as anyone else with a newborn child. It would be over time that I learned she had autism. It was one of many things I learned about her.

Two clues stand out to me now from those first days. One, she became amazing at nursing, but only after a very rough start. Once a specialist came in and broke the steps down, there was no problem. Before that, it was an incredible struggle and she was inconsolable. I think it reflects a great deal about how she learns today. Once the steps are laid out, she is masterful. Another clue was that I could not hold her too much in certain ways without overstimulating her. All I wanted to do was hold her but she seemed to need some space. She liked better to lie across a pillow on my lap. We spent hours that way. Any change made her inconsolable and very fussy. She was already larger than life, my Caroline, ready to rock our world.

The nurses made it hard to feel good about myself in those first moments. I felt the hardest struggle was having outsiders judge as Caroline fussed. I heard many criticisms about how it didn't seem like motherhood came naturally to me, that being older (35) I must be less flexible about what to do, and that "we didn't have books with instructions in our day". Sleepless nights made it harder to take. On top of it, was a mountain-load of advice. Usually not asked for! No matter how polite I was, people didn't leave me alone when I needed it. I loved every minute of being Caroline's mom, being a mom to both Caroline and my second daughter, Emily, but found those early years very hard.

Some people think I am very brave and very confident. However, underneath it all, I am always unsure and looking for someone's approval. I had to simplify the outer world, focus more carefully on the family and the home, and coach myself to have an iron will, and a thick coat of armour. This was hard. I am an art teacher who loves to live for the moment. Before kids, my husband and I would pick up and go camping and hiking. Life was very carefree. I am messy, creative, and generally very scattered. I remember worrying—if my child ends up having autism, how am I going to ever be organized enough to handle it? Routine-oriented? Ha! It sounds like a joke, but for me, it was a serious thing about myself that I needed to change once the children came.

Growing Concerns

Some people have a challenging baby and it resolves with time. Others, like me, have a baby who one day will have a diagnosis like autism. That was the next stress for me. Wondering. Does she have autism? What should I do if she did?

Awareness about autism spectrum disorder is so common now. The efforts to get parents to seek an early diagnosis and early intervention were very widespread when I was a new mother in 2006. Caroline had autism spectrum disorder from birth, but we did not know that initially. There were many, many inconclusive signs. Most of those showed up with the sleeplessness, periods of crying, some unusual behaviours, and her unconventional speech development. The full diagnosis was not until she was just about three-years-old. This was a difficult time because we did not know what to do. We learned a lot in those days about our sunny baby and toddler who loved to play with balls, turtles, and musical toys.

My husband had a serious health issue and went on medical leave. Caroline went from 6 to 8 to 10 months, and I faithfully checked the list of baby's development given out by the health unit. Home was stressful and when I called in with concerns, often the health unit suggested it was the stress that was affecting Caroline, not an issue with her development. This delayed our concerns a little but I couldn't let it go fully.

She was developing well, just at her own pace. She walked sooner than many toddlers, but did not crawl and did not pull herself up, for example. She eventually stood up on her own at daycare, but they called her "yoga baby". She would press her head on the floor and use it for balance as she got her legs under her. She looked like she was defying the restrictions of her body. It was adorable–and definitely unique.

Then daycare led to new awareness. This was also very, very hard to deal with. We were called in to meet the daycare director. She told us that Caroline's language skills and interaction were in urgent need of more attention. I called our local children's centre, Five Counties, and I was given a resource teacher and placed on the waiting list for speech pathology. I was told it would be at least a year to wait. I felt awful—I am a teacher, and I wasn't doing enough to teach my child how to talk.

I was having a person come to my home to see me and offer "services". I was terrified that a messy kitchen or floor would be judged—were they offering services or checking to see if there were problems in the home? I wish I could go and tell that earlier version of myself that it was okay. If only I could. It's okay to call the government and say your child might have autism—that you need a spot on their waiting list for services. It's okay to go to a hearing centre and test your daughter's hearing because you are worried your child has autism, it's okay to get ear tubes put in. It's okay to let workers come into your house to help you. You don't have to do everything they tell you, but let them come in. It's okay to hope that you are wrong about everything. But it's okay to get help, too.

I had trouble with having therapists. For one reason, I thought I knew what to do because I am a teacher. I didn't. I needed their feedback. That made me cry. For another reason, Caroline didn't say "mom". For all the love I poured into her, she seemed indifferent to the new baby and much warmer to her dad than to me. When a young lady came to work with her on her speech or occupational therapy, she was adoring towards her and seemed to prefer her. This hurt.

I wish I could shake my former self, depressed from lack of sleep, and tell myself to take those much needed breaks—let others share the time with Caroline who was such a joy to them. I know my daughter's love for me is so deep and pure she does not feel it is necessary to show it. She knows she has me wholly and does not need to win me over. And I am her safe place if she feels like she needs someone to be angry or sad with. If I could go back now, I would be unapologetic about any sink full of dishes or laundry on the couch. I would get right into it and accept the help offered without feeling ashamed or scared. And I would have done something early about my depression. It is common enough, even without the pressures of raising a child with special needs. I loved my years with my little ones, but they took their toll on my physical and mental health.

I have no regrets for the choices I made in those early years. I accepted help, called the agencies, got on waiting lists. Waits are long. You cannot count on services being available when you need them, but you must find as many resources as you can and advocate for them. Then, ride it out while you wait. Many people told me they refused to put their names on the list because they were not sure. This delays your chance to get treatment if you do end up needing it. I am proud that I had the courage to make the call to Autism Ontario "just in case" when Caroline was 15-months-old.

We gathered as much information as possible. We got a little therapy to help us get started. I fumbled. Visual schedules, countdown clocks, reward system. I am not really organized and just felt like this added to our chaos. Transitions, songs, and five minute warnings are all fine and well until you have to tell Caroline to get out of the pool or leave the playground. A lot of them didn't work. What worked was being firm, holding our own, and not giving in. Being busy and spending time together. Playing games. Singing songs. And watching TV while eating goldfish. Breaks were important, too.

Speech Pathology

Magical things happened when I got help. Therapy can be amazing! Here is just one example. My speech pathologist, Ellen, told me to give Caroline choices—obvious ones, like a cookie or a piece of broccoli. I had to wait until she said cookie, full and loud, before she got it. I made attempts every hour for three days. She screamed and cried. I felt like a horrible, horrible person waving a cookie in front of a toddler and not giving it to her. It is an awful experience to be sure, so I must add that I gave her plenty of other food choices during this time and made sure she felt safe and loved.

Then she said it—cookie. She did it! She got three. She devoured them (oh, she still has a great appetite, the doctors at the time called her a "magnificent specimen"). Then she laughed—a full, deep bellied laugh, sounding out "hahaha", walked up to me and said "cookie". I gave her one more. More laughter resounded in the house and more words. Within a week, she was using over 80 words.

Every time she requested something, she got it. This intense level of reward faded after a while. The language stayed. Now she is 13, and I have to say, she is much better at asking for things than hearing no. She is strong-willed and persistent.

I can honestly say I am not proud of withholding a cookie from a toddler, but it has only done good in the long run. I became stronger that day. I learned that I could do something, I didn't just have to witness meltdowns and handle problems. And it showed me that therapy worked. I also learned that it was up to myself and my husband. Therapists might give you programming or feedback, but they do not do all of the implementation. They teach you. You do it. And you can do that work as much as you choose, based on what feels right. I threw myself into using ABA strategies, visual schedules, and additional educational opportunities to modify behavior and build skills. But at the same time, we took breaks when and where we needed it.

Diagnosis Confirmed

We had bad news along with the great strides we were making. I think in those days I thought we could save her from the autism diagnosis and cure her challenges. There really isn't a cure, but there are chances to maximize the potential. Part of it requires therapists, and they require your own money or government funding. The A-DOS test gives an autism diagnosis and that diagnosis gave us the funding. This was very, very heartbreaking to go through.

The day the resource teacher, Lynne, came to my house while my two girls were asleep. She didn't stay long. Just long enough to say she was recommending Caroline for the ADOS (Autism Diagnostic Observation Schedule) test. I am shaky and crying just remembering that day. It couldn't be true. It wasn't real. And even though I see it now, at the time I didn't fully believe what we had was really autism in my daughter. She insisted we should move forward and start to accept the truth.

When she left, I just wanted my mom. But my mom couldn't save me from this. I had to accept it and handle the results of that test. I put a blanket tightly around my shoulders and sat near a sunny window. I shivered even though it was so warm. I called my husband and told him. I was there to support him while he registered the news–then each of our parents—whose reactions were very emotional and mixed up, as well. This was painful and I grieved along with others. And yet, I had to explain things over and over. It took an incredible toll.

At the time, there was a lot of funding for children with the autism diagnosis. Although other parents were relieved their child was not going to be placed on the spectrum, it ended up giving me more resources and support than I would have had otherwise. I had to go through with it, I had to take it. Then figure out what I had to do.

After breaking the news to my husband, we told the grandparents (we have six in that role). Each responded differently. All needed to understand it. They visited and wanted to talk about it. One conflict that we had was that it was difficult and complicated to explain. We wanted to be supportive to our parents, but we couldn't always answer their questions. Their knowledge of disabilities widely ranged because it was different in the past generations. After many visits with long, drawn out conversations, we realized Caroline was upset. She understood enough to believe that people weren't happy with her. These discussions ended right then and there, and we put her needs first. It left our elders to figure things out on their own. We decided family time was as "autism-free" as possible and we would just enjoy the time together.

I know it sounds like all I went through were these awful experiences—and believe me, watching your toddler do a behavioural test through a one-way mirror window is horrendous—but the best thing that happened to us was getting that out in the open. No more wondering. Just deciding what to do from there. And in between, so much love and joy. My children and I played endlessly. These were some of the best years of my life.

Ups and Downs

The next phase of motherhood I remembered following the diagnosis, was getting Caroline started in school, trying to move on and get things going for her. Many decisions had to be made. I remember finding it strange to get a child ready for kindergarten. Numbers, letters, shapes, potty training. We had an occupational therapist help us regularly at this time. Actually, just after Caroline's diagnosis, we had the pediatrician, speech pathologist, resource teacher, and two occupational therapists; a lot of adults working with a tiny little preschooler. We'd go from meetings, to looking at her innocently drawing or looking at a book. So innocent, and so little. All this fuss for itty bitty her! It seemed excessive.

I tried very hard to keep life going as normal. Socially, there weren't play dates (not really, anyway) and outings were limited by appointments and therapy. I persisted to enjoy life as much as I could. When I tried to do things, I was often in over my head. I heard over and over, as Caroline melted down and Emily joined her in crying too, "we all have those days". But I wanted to cry. For me it was every day! I felt like I couldn't do anything right. I tried though. Trips to the zoo, the pool, relatives, and friends' houses, shopping. Something inside me told me that if I persisted, I would get her used to it, then we would get to do more.

When there was crying at the supermarket, restaurant, or store, my girls often got little treats and gifts. I worried that this reinforced it and kept the crying loud. But it's hard to refuse! Once, they were given a gift in an extremely kind gesture. It's a lovely story. One lady gave each of my girls, screaming and crying at the Swiss Chalet restaurant a teddy bear. She had made them by hand and was giving them out to kids who needed them. Each bear was beautiful and dressed up in a little skirt and had jewelry. That day, the lady wanted us to have the bears, so we would know it was fine if we tried to go out even though it was hard. I'll never forget that kindness.

Sometimes when I was out doing something, I was stuck. The girls would be inconsolable when I had no way to get them home quickly. Once, at a swimming pool, a lady had to hold Emily while I got Caroline dressed. She never liked leaving the water and was crying angrily. Another time, berry picking, I needed help on a tractor. Caroline was in a total meltdown in the middle of a field. We had to take the tractor back. She needed someone to hold her because the noise terrified her, but Emily needed help as well. Caroline screamed and cried for three hours in a meltdown after that, only calming down by zipping herself into a lifejacket and falling asleep. When we visited friends, she often had meltdowns. I can't count the number of times my husband or I would visit alone while the other drove her around. She could not cope with going into someone's home and not knowing what to expect.

It was hard. We had to simplify our lives. We stayed home more. It was hard to go out. Some friends disappeared while others understood and supported us. We built up slowly to doing the things we used to love. Joel broke it down into steps, even driving up to a campground three hours away to set up without any anxiety or tantrums, so that Caroline would understand camping.

We kept at it and I now take both girls swimming, hiking, into Toronto—everywhere—but I had to push through those early years and get Caroline accustomed to being out, transitioning to and from the activity, coming home again.

And I can say it all paid off. We camp, hike in mountains, swim in the ocean, skate, ski, and ride bikes with her. She gets into activities like a speed skating club which has been amazing with her. We take road trips weeks on end, and she loves it. When we are home, she spends lots of her time looking joyfully at our pictures.

Decisions

I began to think I was causing problems by using daycare, continuing to work, and trying to do all the things other children do in our free time. I debated quitting teaching and homeschooling Caroline. One pediatrician told me to take her situation much more seriously. But he also told me, "You are not a therapist, you are her mother. You need to be her mother. Don't quit your job. Just take your job as her mother seriously."

I cried at that. I was serious about motherhood. If anything, I was too intense and had to deal with my own anxiety and depression. It was not post-partum, I learned that for sure. And my situation intensified it. I got myself straightened out, and kept my job which helped my mental health a great deal. I get a lot of joy out of teaching art. Financially, looking ahead, it was probably a good idea to keep the pension and benefits.

I decided to stop apologizing for the choices I made. I became a better mother when I stopped second-guessing myself. I loved coming home from work and being with my girls. I owe my vice principal and my principals for their support in the ups and downs of raising a child with special needs. There were a few leaves and reduced schedules, and more than a few messy days because I had to leave. I learned to forgive myself and to look forward.

Choices to work or not work are often made for you. If I left my job, I'd never get it back. It really wasn't a choice. Others find work and childcare unaffordable, or prefer to stay home. These are all good choices, and as I said, they are so often made for you. Don't fret over it.

School and the IBI Program

I don't want to paint a rosy picture of what came after. I feel Caroline at 13-years-old is a sharp, clever character with incredible life skills and an amazing knack for communication. We made it through the system and she got a great deal out of it. We benefited from school and the IBI program that Autism Ontario recently cancelled. But by no stretch of the imagination did she get everything she needed. We hated much about the system and worked hard to make up for its shortcomings ourselves.

The year Caroline started kindergarten, I had an IEP meeting with 19 people all advocating for an EA for her. It was an excessive amount of people. In the end, we were only guaranteed support in the school for a short time, while she got used to kindergarten. We managed to stretch it out through kindergarten and into Grade 1. One year, the principal pulled the EA out because the needs in the school were so high; she didn't feel Caroline had enough challenging behaviours. That teacher said she couldn't find time for Caroline and could not teach her. I screamed and yelled the day I found out. I am not proud of my behavior. It got us nowhere. Caroline often got put on the side of the room and left to her own worksheets while the rest of the class learned. In subsequent years, while she had IBI, there was finally support for her autism, but she missed two years of school. We couldn't win. But between school, IBI, and our own efforts, we got through it all.

We took things on for ourselves. School became her social opportunity to be around others and get more interaction. At home, she insisted on a shower, pyjamas, and then the reading and math would begin. We'd go into the school, show the teacher she could read—the teacher didn't even know! It got us nowhere. In our school system, unless you have dangerous behavior, you don't get direct support. Being able to learn is not enough to generate the funding. It's horrible and makes us very angry. What are we doing when the vulnerable don't get support for an education?

We learned not to have angry discussions at home because Caroline could understand everything. She thought we were unhappy with her. Never! My poor little one. Now that she is older, she is remembering those early days and talking about it. It's incredible what she has been aware of all the time. Not surprisingly, it has made us all very emotional.

Her potential is incredible and she continues to surprise us every day. She is almost done with her timetables, reads well, and is learning to cook. She does chores without being asked. She is such a hardworking, responsible, and resilient person. For everything we went through, she was asked to leave her comfort zone, try new things, and struggle through huge barriers of communication. Most of it happened because of the hours we worked on it all at home, repeating tasks, and breaking things down. But most of it also happened because of how determined and courageous this young girl is in her character.

We have had amazing successes because of her spirit. She has reached the hearts of people in her schools and changed people's minds about what children with disabilities can do. I'll never forget my pride at her Grade 6 graduation, as she walked with the rest of the class, and sat listening attentively to the speeches and awards. She was proud to be there with her class. To our joy and pride, she was given a truly special award, the Sierra Smiles award, in honour of a little girl at the school who lost her life to cancer. Caroline was honoured for her resilience, positive energy, and the joy she brought others at her school.

No matter how many challenges we had, there were also moments like this of unspeakable joy and beauty. The invitation to her EA's wedding. The valentines she gave out to all the children with special needs in the school from kindergarten to Grade 6. Her ability to swing higher than high on the playground. Her smart comments that made the whole class dissolve in laughter when people were having problems. We had a different path in the childhood years but it was fulfilling with many wonderful moments.

Not the End

I am of course very afraid about what her adult life will bring. I am working on learning what I can do to make it better for her. I am reaching out to Community Living, and hoping more answers will come to me. I try to look ahead at least five years so that I can learn as much as I can before it happens. I don't know if it will all be fine, but I'm doing as much as I can.

When I think of my new-mother struggles, I am ashamed of grieving the diagnosis. I have become stronger, more loving, and more resourceful than I ever believed. My marriage is strong, for which I am grateful. If I could tell that artsy, flaky, happy-go-lucky former self how it would end up—I don't know if I'd believe this was me. All I know is that I believed in myself. And I've had joy to equal any pain. If you are reading this, because you are now getting the news that you have a child with special needs, please stay strong when it's rough. Hang on to those golden moments. Never apologize to anyone if you need to work differently through your situation. I wish you the joy and the growth that will happen in the years to come.

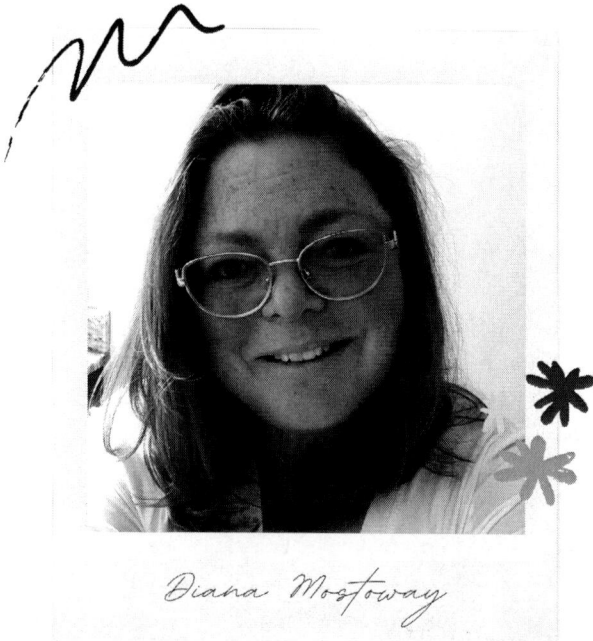

Diana Mostoway

Diana Mostoway is a high school art teacher in Peterborough, Ontario. She has a passion for the outdoors and any creative pursuit. She discovered that her daughter showed signs of being on the autism spectrum when she started her in daycare at just 13-months-old. Now, her daughter is 13 and has made incredible strides, making her say, "never say never". Her key to success has been immense love and zero hesitation to put her name on waitlists or to try out a therapy session for speech, behavior, or occupational therapy. As a family of four, the Mostoways spend their time on the road camping throughout Canada, and visiting several grandparents in their homes across Ontario. School and learning take a high priority, whether it is piano, sport, or mathematics during family time. Her dreams of being a productive artist have been shelved for the time being, but she couldn't be happier.

To Be a Child Is All I Need

By Isabel Neves

My name is Isabel Neves. I was born in a small town in Portugal on September 25th, 1969. We lived a simple life; we survived by working in the fields, growing all kinds of vegetables, and taking care of our farm animals. I remember living off of candle light until electricity reached our village. Our fireplace was used to cook our food. Our alarm clock was the rooster, and since each family had one, no one could sleep through it. The bell at church rang for several reasons, to remind us of the time, if something happened, and to pray three Hail Mary's at 6 a.m., noon, and 6 p.m. We had different sounds for different situations. We celebrated the Holy days with parades, music, dances, and at night we would pray The Rosary together as a family.

Since we only had one doctor in our village, we only went to the doctor to get our vaccinations. It was up to us to live a healthy life by maintaining a healthy body—we only consumed natural and fresh foods. As for my education, I only completed up to Grade 6. We could not afford to stay in school any longer as we are a big family and my parents needed help on the farm. Therefore I found myself involved with my community as the people there became my family. We were always there for each other and available to lend a helping hand. I loved helping the kids from my village with their homework, with prayer and bible study at church, and with community acting performances. Our household was the first to have a telephone and it acted as a community phone. When one person called from outside or needed to call someone, they would come to our house. My older brother and I used to be the messenger. When the government started to charge more taxes and bills began to appear for the telephone, electricity, and taxes for the fields, we went into debt. We could no longer afford to pay the employees that had helped us.

In 1987, my father decided to immigrate to Canada. He brought along one of my brothers and some of his cousins, but the rest of us stayed home. Two years later, around the time I turned nineteen, he brought the whole family with him to Canada. During this time in Canada, construction workers and those in other fields were not being compensated enough for their work; they had to fight for their rights. My father wanted us to go to school, but because of our financial situation, we went to work first. My first job was in a restaurant where I worked from 8 a.m. until 11 p.m. along with my younger sister. I earned $800 per month plus tips. I began to get bad headaches and little to no sleep. I went to the doctor and he told me I was too young to get sleeping pills. He recommended that if I cannot acclimate to this country that I should go back home.

With my working environment at the time and the difference between countries, I was struggling to adapt. However, I refused to go back home because my whole family was now here. I suffered through the migraines and continued working to help support my parents. Eventually I began to get worse. I went to the doctor again and after an examination, he told me I needed to stop smoking, my lungs were not in a good state. However, I had never smoked before. The fumes from the restaurant coupled with people smoking indoors gave me second-hand smoke. I hated it and was so mad. I was getting sick because of other people, and seeing people smoke in the restaurant with kids around every time I served meals killed me inside. It got to the point where I was getting panic attacks and had to quit.

My father told me to go back to school, but I refused. Later in 1998, I got married and a year later, got pregnant. My doctor told me I had to stay home and rest throughout my whole pregnancy because my health condition at that time put me at risk of losing my child. All I could do was try to stay calm and pray. I asked God, "Why me?"

In September of 2000, my baby girl was born and came out healthy and strong. It felt like my life was beginning to change for the better. However, a year later, I woke up one morning and could not feel my legs. A big pain struck in my back. I went to the doctor to get pain pills, the chiropractor, and a masseuse for several years. My masseuse told me I needed to be careful or else I may end up in a wheelchair. My health declined even more as I worked in a factory. The pills I had been taking for seven years now were no longer working anymore as my body became used to them.

My doctor told me I had severe chronic major depression and she gave me antidepressants, pain killers, and antacid pills. I had to quit work for good. In 2011 my husband had to bring me to the hospital. I could not feel my body and felt like I was going to die. The hospital could not find anything wrong and sent me home with more pills. I did not take the pills and quit taking pills in general. I went to my doctor and was sent to do some tests. After an ultrasound, the nurse looked at me and smiled saying, "Congratulations! You are 10 weeks pregnant". I was speechless and confused. I was dealing with tremendous body pain, bitter taste in my tongue and acid in my stomach. Turns out I had a bacteria in my stomach that I could not fix until I gave birth. However, I was so happy at the blessing I had been given.

My son, Ismael, was born on December 18th, 2011. He was diagnosed with autism spectrum disorder when he was three-years-old. I did not understand the meaning of the disability. He was a very healthy boy and very bright in many ways. Everything started when he went to school. He started getting sick, vomiting, and getting fevers. I was getting calls from school to pick him up because of his behaviour. Everytime I gave him medication he got very frustrated and I saw the impact of medication on his behaviour; it made him a different boy. He even told me that the medication kills him. Some of the medications used were puffers, antibiotics, Advil, and Tylenol. I prayed to God for guidance and to give me an answer.

I recalled that in the bible the use of oils for healing was prevalent. I then started using oils from Young Living and everything began to change for good. Not just for my son, but for the whole family. My daughter's allergies slowly disappeared as I began to diffuse oils at home, and my son's demeanor became calmer. Along with using the oils, I switched to using natural products. I changed to organic and whole foods and it made a huge difference. I stopped giving him medication and there were no more calls from school. Instead, he completed his academic work and he was happy because of the friends he began to make. As a parent I am very proud of my child and very happy I found the oils. We are not alone. Our children will be the adults of tomorrow. God is the creator of all good things. It is up to us to accept and use it and be grateful everyday.

I have been volunteering to help the students at school and involved in Adara's Foundation. I have met beautiful people along the way. Dr. Sabina Devita has been an amazing doctor as she gives me the oils and supplements I need that make a difference in my health, and the health of my children. She has helped me in my emotional and spiritual healing as well. I can now see how God works in mysterious ways and God has blessed people like Gary Young to aid us along the way.

To Be a Child is All I Need
Time and freedom to love and receive love.
Time and freedom to learn to understand
The world around me.
Time and freedom with somebody who can
Trust and understand me.

Time and freedom to grow up hours, minutes
and different kinds of weathers.
The best thing I need in this world in order
to be a child is time, understanding and to
be free.
Love all children
The children of today are the adults of
tomorrow.

—By Isabel Neves

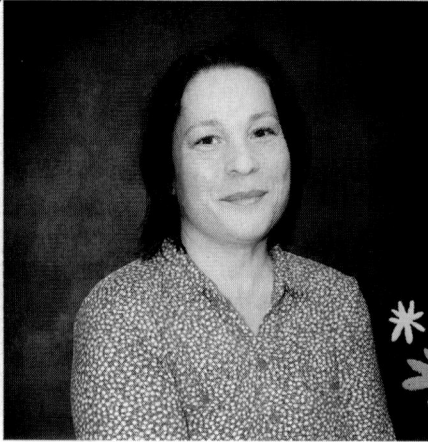

Isabel Neves

Isabel Neves is a work-from-home parent by choice who takes care of her family. She is a mother of two children, one diagnosed with autism spectrum disorder (ASD). In her free time, she volunteers with a non-profit organization called Adara's Foundation. This foundation aims to support families with children diagnosed with ASD. She enjoys forming these connections with families and to help support their needs. Isabel also spends her time volunteering at school and being a substitute teacher. As an extroverted person, she can often be found outdoors with family and friends, or gardening. She is an advocate for healthy living which has led to her working with Young Living Essential Oils to spread awareness for an alternative lifestyle. She loves to spend time outdoors with her friends and family, and gardening.

Email: isabelneves813@gmail.com

When the Screaming Stops

By Sonia Regan

He wet the bed again. It's a familiar routine for us these days. He wakes us, his clothes soaking in urine, the smell strong enough to rouse even the deepest sleep. I take him to the shower, coax him to take off his clothes and run the water for him. Physically, he can do it himself, but he needs constant guidance and supervision to know what to do. I lay out his clothes on his bed, coach him out of the running water and help him dry his adult-sized, man-body. He is not a little boy anymore. He towers over me with his ever-increasing body hair and strength. I use the opportunity to talk to him about protective behaviours. To tell him it is not okay for others to touch his private parts or to see him naked and I try to encourage him to dry his own body. In my own head, I just hope he never has to draw on these words, to remember what mum told him about being touched. But, I know the risks for him are higher than they are for others.

He has been pacing all morning. Wandering the length of the house, his steps becoming more pronounced. He is repeating phrases from movies and television shows he enjoys. But his voice is becoming louder, faster, and less coherent. There is a kind of angry tone to his voice, although there is no apparent reason for him to be angry.

I offer him breakfast and he shakes his wrist to indicate positively. He rarely says yes or no anymore and prefers to sign. I make him his preferred cereal and pour juice into the plastic purple cup, the only cup he will use. I have barely put everything away before he indicates he has finished. Again, he chooses to use sign language, rather than interrupt his increasingly pervasive verbal torrent.

He is stomping now and producing a deep-throated scream that sounds as though he is being tortured. I hear my husband say something about the neighbours calling the police, but I don't react. His whole body is tense, each muscle tightened. His eyes are wide open, and his pupils are dilated. But he won't look at me. His eyes dart around the room, not looking at anything in particular, but taking in everything.

I stay nearby but am wary of the risks he poses to me. He is taller, heavier, and stronger than me now. I have a flashback to when he was younger, and I tried to stop him banging his head against a wall. I rub my cheekbone as I remember the blackeyes and bruises he had given me when I was less careful. I keep my voice lowered but I know he can't hear it over his loud, blood-curdling screams. I speak softly and try to maintain contact with him as a reminder that I am with him. I stroke his arm gently and he grabs my hand tightly, digging in his nails and squeezing so tightly I wonder what it would take to break my fingers.

It's hard to look calm when your insides are falling apart. It's hard to look your child in the eye and try to reassure them that the world is not the scary, unpredictable place they think it is; to reassure him I am here for him and can be bigger and stronger and make the world a safe, secure place for him. It is exhausting. I take a deep breath and hope the screaming will stop soon.

I ask him to take deep breaths with me. I don't honestly expect him to respond but I hold up my hands to indicate we will count 10 breaths. He pushes my hands away and screams a little louder. My ears are ringing and my heart is pounding but I raise my hands again. He looks at me and takes a single deep breath. Then, pushes me aside to continue pacing the length of the house.

He is hot. The high levels of adrenaline seem to elevate his body temperature, even though it is a cool summer day. I grab a wet cloth and he allows me to touch it to his face and neck. The yelling continues but at least he is now sitting next to me on the couch. I manage to get him to take 10 deep breaths. I breathe with him. It isn't enough to lower my adrenaline, but it helps.

The yelling begins to ease. He continues to repeat movie phrases, but he appears slightly more relaxed. He turns and looks me in the eye. I smile. It is a genuine smile because the screaming has stopped, but it is also for his benefit—to remind him I am still here, no matter what.

As I sit next to him, I watch as his body begins to relax. His jaw unclenches and his eyes relax. He points to his eyes and I wonder to myself if this is the first time he has blinked in the last hour. I stroke his forehead gently and give him permission to rest his eyes if he needs to. He motions for me to follow him to the kitchen. There is a calendar on the fridge with his school holiday schedule carefully mapped out. There is almost a full month of uncrossed days staring back at me. He points to the end of the month where I have scrawled "back to school". And I realise he is lost. He doesn't know how to initiate play or create his own fun. And he is bored.

He is tired. The high levels of adrenaline have drained him and he points to his bed. I help him climb in and encourage him to rest. He doesn't resist. I close the door and go to find my husband. He wraps his arms around me, knowingly. We have been here many times before, and we both know we will be there again. I feel single tears roll down my cheeks as I let go of the strong exterior.

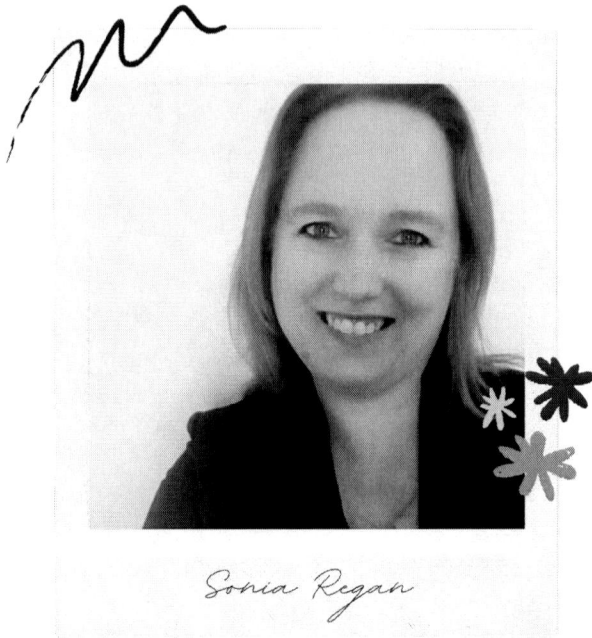

Sonia Regan

Sonia is a parent of a young adult with an intellectual disability and autism spectrum disorder. She has lived and worked in community development and disability for almost 20 years. Sonia is well recognised for her passion for empowering communities and families to navigate services with confidence. Sonia runs an awareness blog on Facebook—A is for Aysh, where she shares her experiences with disability in the home and community.

Website: www.soniaregan.com

Comfort and Growth Never Co-exist

By Laurie and Joe Sehl

If you are reading this book because you have a child with special needs, feel blessed. It's the most challenging and amazing growth experience the universe could have given you. You'll see!

In 1999, our son Grant was diagnosed with PDD-NOS at three-years-old (pervasive development disorder - not otherwise specified). In today's terms, we would recognize this as ASD (autism spectrum disorder). Back then, autism was often compared to Dustin Hoffman's character in *Rainman*. "Would Grant really turn out like Rainman?" we wondered. How naïve we were, and so was the rest of society at that time. This chapter reflects on our learning through Grant who is now 24-years-old. We hope this helps you.

The Diagnosis

We learned that our son may have more than a speech delay about 15 minutes into our first speech therapy appointment. Right away, our therapist said we should have him assessed. Luckily for us, that same office had various child professionals who all worked together, and we were quickly referred to the child psychologist for assessment. A private assessment of Grant was a very good decision based on hindsight. We had benefits that partially covered the costs. It still was expensive, but worth it. We found the advantages to be many.

a) First, by employing our own team of professionals, we could call on them when we felt we needed them. Sure it cost, but this was our child and we knew the first six years were critical so we spent the money and didn't regret it.

b) We avoided the long wait times for assistance in the education system.

c) We had control over who saw his assessment and could get a copy any time we needed it for tax purposes etc. A disability tax credit was significant.

d) We had the same people reviewing Grant's progress over time, even into his young adulthood. That was huge for Grant. He had a psychologist and a speech therapist who worked in conjunction. They knew him, truly cared about him, and could see his progress over time and make intelligent recommendations. They encouraged us when we needed it and gave us a little kick in the butt when we got lazy. This

111

same team was involved in his initial diagnosis, again when starting elementary school, then high school, and finally university. Yes, he is graduating from Medical Physics at Ryerson University, Toronto in the fall of 2020. We are so proud of him.

If Grant's therapists are still practicing (my little group of angels) we'll likely get their advice as he joins the work world. We can't say enough about these people who need to be acknowledged, Lynda Rowden and Associates who also included Paul Moss, his early years speech therapist based in Brampton, Ontario.

Telling Grant about his Diagnosis

It was a tough decision. We decided, based on our research, that telling Grant about his diagnosis sooner than later was preferred. It was a memorable experience. We asked him if he knew what autism was. His response was telling. He said, "Is it a society?" He was eight-years-old, very intelligent, and observant. He read mail coming into the house from the Autism Society of Ontario, hence his response.

In our discussion about Grant's diagnosis, we included some famous people who were thought to be autistic (Einstein, Glen Gould, Dan Acroyd) and explained how gifted they were and how their minds worked differently than most people. We told him that these gifted people sometimes have a hard time in certain situations like getting upset easily (we further described some of Grant's challenges). He then asked, "Am I autistic?" We said yes, we think so. To our surprise, he was quite proud of his diagnosis. It couldn't have been a better outcome.

Even today, Grant embraces his link to this world of autism and refers to himself as an Aspie. He often says, "We aspies have a hard time understanding you sometimes". It's amazing. Grant has a friend on the spectrum who is currently touring as a comedian. Check out Michael McCreary at www.aspiecomic.com. He's another inspiration you can draw on.

Support Services

The support team mentioned above gave us valuable insights into the resources at our disposal through the government and elsewhere. Admittedly, we didn't use them as much as we could have. We were blessed with close family and with good incomes, so we didn't feel we should take someone else's spot for respite care, etc. We did however get support from Caledon Community Services who offered special in-home council which was helpful, and they introduced us to "play therapy".

Play therapy at three-years-old turned out to be a great break for us but also an opportunity for Grant to socialize with kids like himself. It was rough, there were lots of tantrums, but the therapists were patient. We think it helped him move forward at a time when we were in a fog of figuring out what to do.

Support Tools

Back in 1999, we relied on our speech therapist heavily for ideas on how to support Grant at home. It turned out, we were the best therapists Grant could have had because we knew him so well and spent the most time with him. The danger was that we put too much pressure on ourselves, and also had a tough time balancing quality time with his older brothers who felt neglected and resentful. We recommend that parents should be prepared to skip a therapy session or invest in a trusted college student to babysit while you take time for yourselves, your other kids, your spouse and friends. It's better in the end. Respite resources would have been perfect for this.

Some really great tools that helped us included:

- Books by Temple Grandin—There are thousands of books about autism now, but back then, they were geared to professionals. We didn't have time to read them all and found them too technical. Out of the gate, we found Temple Grandin's books about her personal journey as a person with autism extremely helpful. I found her to be the most credible and helpful resource to help us understand our son. *Talking in Pictures* (her book and now a movie) offered fascinating insight for the whole family blessed with a nonverbal child with ASD. Temple tours has an active website (www.templegrandin.com) and has other resources available (TED Talks, etc). I highly recommend spending some time with her material and/or seeing her speak in person.

- Pictures or PECs—We started trying to help Grant speak with this tool. He was nonverbal until he started using some words at about four or five-years-old, gradually got more verbal over time. Of interest: when Grant did become more verbal, he moved quickly to full sentences. He wasn't verbal but must have been forming full sentences in his mind.

- Social Stories—This was huge for us. You can buy social story books through your speech therapist but you can also just create your own. Social stories are "teaching stories". Grant loved to listen to bedtime stories so we leveraged that to our advantage. We would create our own little book with words and hand drawn pictures about a lesson we wanted him to learn. Grant's older brother was his nemesis and best teacher. They are friends now, but it was a challenge for a long time. Social stories really helped with that.

- Overnight Camp—Yes, Grant went to camp twice for one week each time. He was great and had a blast, but we didn't enter into it lightly. We were freaked out to say the least but had friends sending their child to the same camp which gave us some comfort. We took the time to consider Grant's challenges and made sure the camp was willing to take a child on the spectrum. We took a great deal of time to document Grant's behaviours and sensitivities so that the people supporting him had a good chance of helping him when he needed it. We talked to them over the phone and gave them our contact numbers in case there were questions or problems. Grant is a very confident kid despite his challenges, in part due to his experiences away from home throughout his childhood.

- The Boundless School—This was an interesting journey and an incredible experience for Grant. In short, it was an outdoor education experience where he earned a high school credit. He camped in the wilderness (supervised) in the Ottawa Valley. We were freaked out for the whole week, but it peaked when Grant (terrified of thunderstorms) was camping during a reported tornado. The campers learned quickly how to trench around their tents so they didn't get flooded. The counselor had to hang out with Grant during the really tough part of the storm, but man, talk about conquering his fears! There was never a problem with thunderstorms since.

- Drama lessons—Drama lessons were huge for Grant. One wise teacher in highschool recommended that Grant take drama in Grade 10. Her theory was that if Grant doesn't naturally know how to be social he could mimic being social by using acting skills. Yes, fake it. It turned out to be the best thing ever. Grant took drama all through the remainder of highschool and during university. Drama classes were Grant's safe place to be himself and practice his skills. In fact, Grant graduated from the Second City Academy of Arts, and now can try out for main stage events. He made friends, found his sense of humour, built great confidence and has a hobby for life. His Second City troop's last show and finale included Grant singing a solo that he wrote himself, about feeling awkward around other people and how he overcame it with friends like the people in his second city troop. It was one of the most emotional points of this amazing journey for us. The tears flowed for a good hour after that, confusing the heck out of Grant. There is another lesson here; that is one of talent. If you have a child on the spectrum you will often hear that your child will have "deficits" and "talents". Things they do not do well (often social interaction) but things they do very well. And the key is to find the things they do very well and build on those, while minimizing the gaps. I think there is tremendous truth here but also be wary of expectations that the child will have genius-like talents. In Grant's case, he has a terrific memory (for things that interest him), he's an excellent mimic. And despite being challenged in social settings where he is not familiar, he's somewhat fearless in front of an audience. Is it genius level? No. But it is a talent that he can celebrate.

- Sports—Grant had to trial several sports before he landed on a few he really resonated with. Baseball seemed to stick. He plays baseball even still in the summers with the company team at his summer job and holds his own. We had to be patient and coach him through some temper tantrums when he got frustrated, but it was worth it. Baseball was slower paced than traditional hockey or lacrosse teams. Baseball is also a game of rules. Grant appreciates rules, especially when they are enforced. This is not uncommon. In all things, we found consistency and following rules helped Grant. In sports, we found Brampton Special Needs Hockey, part of SHI (Special Hockey International), was an amazing way to give Grant the team experience in a loving and understanding environment. They support any child with mental disabilities who can stand up on ice. Grant started at eight-years-old and continues to participate in this organization at 23-years-old. He loves it. Special Olympics we never experienced, but many friends did and loved it.

Our final recommendation is to take an active role in your child's life, school, and therapy. You can then learn from the professionals and then practice at home. Take the time to educate the rest of your family as well. The more you work together, the less pressure you will feel as a parent. Our family was always interested in helping if we took the time to educate them (easier said than done). Take care of yourself. It's the "oxygen first on the airplane" theory. You can't help your child if you are stressed or overwhelmed. It sounds selfish, but it's not!

From a Father's Perspective

This is Grant's dad's recollection of determining Grant was on the spectrum and some miscellaneous thoughts for others: as I recall, we felt there were some delays in Grant's development, but thought it was more to do with him being a member of a busy family with two older brothers that did his talking for him. It wasn't until a babysitter raised this issue, using the term autism specifically, that it caused us to raise our level of concern. And, more frankly for me, to wake up to a reality that I was denying. That evening, I did what many do: I googled. This is dangerous as there is a lot of disinformation out there. But I did come across useful questionnaires, from reputable sources (i.e. Autism Society), that can be used to determine if you should take steps for getting professional advice. I knew that evening that we needed to get help. And I finally understood that autism does not equal *Rainman*.

We were fortunate in that very good friends of ours had a child with special needs and could advise us regarding professionals that could help. Despite all the support we received, I recall being very disillusioned that there was not a specific roadmap provided as to "how to fix this". Today, there is a much greater awareness of the autism diagnosis and of support structures available. But, to be clear, it is a *spectrum*. No one individual is the same as the other. Someone else's experience will not be yours. There is no perfect roadmap. There is no "fix". It's cliché to say, but it is a journey. Take the wins as they come. Do not get down on yourself if you're not feeling blessed everyday. Take care of yourself. Hopefully our experience can help spark ideas for you. I do hope that, in the long run, you experience the blessing that we have received.

Grant has expanded my mind and made me a better person. And for that, I am blessed.

 Laurie and Joe Sehl are from Caledon, Ontario and have been residents there for many years. They are the parents of three boys, Jeffrey—30, Christophe—27, and Grant—24. Currently, Laurie and Joe are sales professionals in the tech industry. Laurie has a keen interest in helping others and is currently completing her fourth level of Healing Touch while Joe is receiving Healing Touch treatments. It's their goal to use their experience and certification in Healing Touch, along with the support of essential oils, to volunteer in hospice, hospitals, and old age homes when in their retirement years.

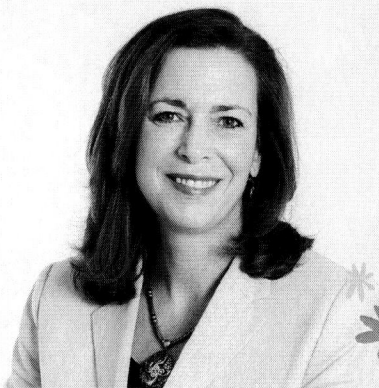

Laurie Sehl

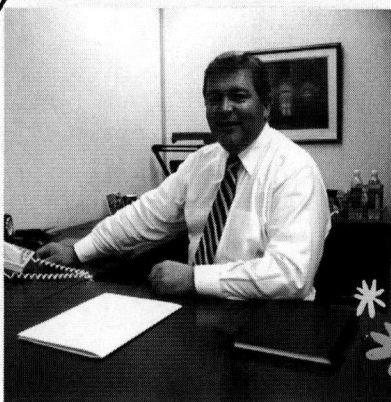

Joe Sehl

Email: laurie.sehl@gmail.com and jpsehl3@gmail.com
LinkedIn: https://www.linkedin.com/in/laurie-sehl-0642b14/
Facebook: Laurie Sehl

There Is No Normal

By Helen Snell

I remember like yesterday hearing the murmurs of the nurses as they hovered over my daughter. I had just delivered my third child. My eyes locked with my husband's and we knew. I rolled my head in their direction from my bed and calmly asked if she had down syndrome. I thought the nurse might drop her. Apologetically, realizing we had overheard, she responded to not be alarmed, and that they were just discussing some features they observed.

I knew. I just knew. We had some genetic markers show up during my pregnancy but chose not to undergo any invasive procedures to confirm. We had chosen Sarah as her name. But something told me that day Victoria would be more fitting since she would rise above and not become her label. Victoria, in the book of baby names, means "victorious". That was also the first day the mask was ripped off the world, humanity softened, and my eyes saw truth.

When I was a young child I used to play "school" with my older siblings. As they grew up I became the teacher for my dolls. I dreamt of being a teacher when I grew up. The twists and turns of life and career landed me far from that profession, but I was always drawn into positions where I could educate and help others. Now was my chance to teach in a new and unique way. Every task with Tori (we shortened her name) had to be broken down into the smallest components for her to grasp. It was a challenge I delighted in. Every milestone was a celebration. Each day a blessing.

We had access to some pretty good help through our local health services regarding development with fine and gross motor skills, feeding, sign language, and early speech. We received referral after referral to groups for support, for programming, and playgroups all in the down syndrome world, and all fairly far from home.

There was this fun little personality developing. Someone who, by the age of two, could put a VCR tape in the machine and turn it on. Someone funny and carefree. Someone who adored her older siblings, and who brought peace and simplicity to our home. Someone who radiated love. We had our share of pity, inappropriate comments, and even discomfort and fear from friends and acquaintances. And we had people try to help by telling us what all down syndrome kids were like. Like the armour of Achilles, or the bubble conjured by Violet Incredible, we were impervious through the love that surrounded our little girl. It was a conscious decision not to attend or join any of these specific DS groups.

I wanted Tori to grow up to be her own person, not labeled by her disability, but known for her unique personality. I used to refer to my experience on our walks and adventures as using my "Tori Vision" because she embraced the world so differently. There was a clarity and focus around her, a simplicity. She also taught us boundaries, honesty, and patience because she didn't have the normal social filters. She would refuse hugs. She would state out loud if she didn't like someone (and she was a pretty good judge of character). She melted the hearts of those who were uncomfortable with her from past experiences or misinformation. Because we let her.

We were fortunate to have a church family where Tori was able to love and be loved. This safe community allowed us to give her this freedom. It allowed her to heal those who were broken. She had a particularly significant relationship with a recovering alcoholic who could not resist her unbiased love. She was the person (little as she was) who made him feel comfortable in the community there. She was a solid rung on the ladder of his life. And our faith community helped her gain confidence to help her transition to school. She was confident and connected to other students her age, and to those who were friends with her older siblings. She was social, loved costumes, and music, memorizing (most) of her first pop song at age six, and performing her first lip-sync in front of an audience around the age of eight.

Over the years I did a lot of research into down syndrome and became familiar with autism as well, eventually certifying for level one autism. Much of this was for my own knowledge, but I did work a few summers at a local volunteer organization. I enjoyed my time working with other children with special needs and grew to quickly see that every child is unique. Successful ABA therapy for one child didn't work for another, aggression was often actually a frustration, and, for Tori, in particular, anxiety was often due to triggers from other children. Many other children in the specialized camps either didn't verbalize their discomfort, or weren't affected by it. Not Tori. Programs for special needs soon weren't working for her.

Tori was integrated into regular gymnastics classes, and town camp programs when she was a bit older. She often fit in with kids a few years younger, and being small in stature, she didn't stand out. Program coordinators were so helpful to provide the support needed. She eventually moved into private gymnastics lessons where she thrived for several years until she declared, "I can do a somersault and a cartwheel. I think I'm done." So she was finished. She had satisfactorily accomplished what she felt was enough.

We took many cues like this from Tori instead of forcing her into programs or behaviours we thought were best. She resisted swimming as a baby but decided around age six she was going to learn to swim, leading to a few summers in constant water wings and life jackets because she had no fear of the water. This translated into theatre, football, and making videos, and now as she is preparing to enter the workforce. She knows what she does and doesn't want to do.

Her very first work placement in high school was at a library where she catalogued books with brilliant success. This played into her organization and slight obsessive-compulsive tendencies. She surprised us the most with her choice to clean tables in the food court at our local mall. I felt this was beneath her abilities, but allowing her to be the guide, we soon discovered it was the social component of the work she loved. She saw friends from school and neighbours out shopping. Some other family friends working in the mall even had lunch with her on occasion. She took great pride in that placement because she was often shown appreciation and kindness from mall patrons for her work.

She has had her share of challenges. She has fears and phobias. She loves intensely and feels such heartbreak when separated from friends or family. She has anxiety and she still often cries as a young adult when things don't quite go her way. She really struggled when we moved to a new town midway through secondary school. The first month she was withdrawn, tearful, and we had to switch some classes around because she couldn't cope at the same academic level as her previous school. This was a setback I wasn't expecting. She had always been confident and social, but I realized she always had allies around her, and this was all new territory. She was fortunate enough to meet a beautiful soul who invited her to participate as the water girl on the boy's football team. This changed everything.

In school she performed in dance recitals and Christmas plays. She integrated herself into all areas throughout her school career. She played with classmates at elementary school recess and had friends over for birthday parties. I realize we were lucky. I know it isn't that easy for most. But I also believe our decision to let Tori be herself relieved us of worry that then did not manifest in her. We could see from an early age she was a free spirit. Other children we met over the years with down syndrome had varied personalities. They could be shy, angry, or even aggressive. I recall an incident in Grade 7 when she was being bullied by a classmate who also had DS. There was a tension in their friendship that sometimes became physical due to the other girl's frustration. Tori has always been a rule follower and tried very hard to be a good student. I told her if her classmate hurt her she had my permission to hit her back, hard. "Let her know you won't put up with it and she will stop." Tori advised us under no circumstances could she hit another student at school. I encouraged her over several conversations to consider it was self-defense. Later that year she kicked a boy in the schoolyard who was playfully teasing her. When a teacher intervened she told them her mom said it was okay. I had to explain the miscommunication, but that was a sure sign to me she understood the basics of boundaries.

But, it was also a realization that her other friend, although very close in intellectual and cognitive delays, was really nothing at all like Tori. There is no down syndrome behavior pattern. There is no common personality trait. You often hear all DS kids are affectionate, or simple, chubby, sedentary, or lack motivation. However, there was no predicted outcome. There was no "abnormal". There was no "normal".

Tori is a tomboy. She is a tech prodigy. She can't do math to save her life. She hovers between wanting to be Justin Bieber and wanting to marry him. She fixes the settings on my phone. She is obstinate. She loves Subway sandwiches and potato chips. And she is terrified of Hallowe'en. Her room is immaculate. But she can't carry a plate to the kitchen counter. She is learning sign language for fun. She is a Special Olympics swimmer. She can do the butterfly stroke. She can't trim her own fingernails. She is my hero.

But this isn't your child. Their behaviors are their own. This understanding was so helpful for me in guiding a friend who gave birth to an awesome boy with down syndrome a few years after Tori was born. And with guiding my other two children through school when they didn't quite fit that mould, either. If we could allow them to be, within a model of safety, we would see their best. If we could take the time to see the world the way they do we could hold space for them in it. We would understand their motivation and use that to teach them to thrive. This isn't different from any other child. Gifted, poor, other needs, or privileged; children are unique and precious. They receive

121

love and show love in their own way. They need their own boundaries and learn in a way unique to each of them. There is no normal behavior, or learning style. There is no standard school curriculum for everyone. There is no special needs, or mainstream. There simply is no normal.

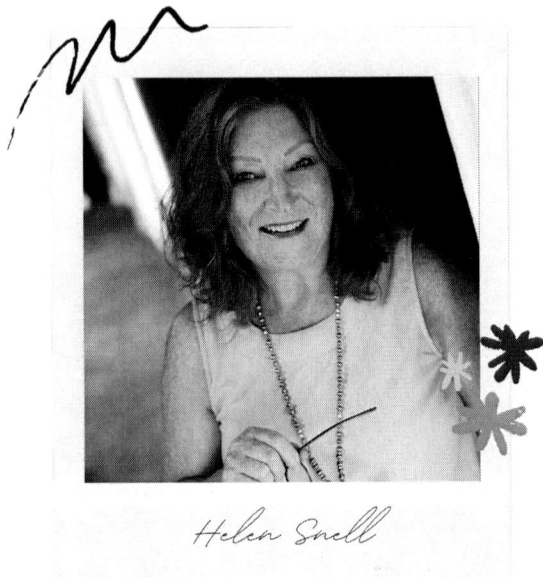

Helen Snell

Helen uses stories to share her passion for sustainable, healthy, and earth-friendly living. She creates stories for others in her business through ghost-writing, blogging, and story brand development. As a brand ambassador for Arbonne, she educates people on healthy choices for their families in vegan skincare and nutrition, and shows them the inspiring way she has connected her passion to her income. She believes strongly in guiding people to take small steps in the right direction for collective impact.

These things revolve around her family of three children, too quickly advancing into adulthood. Her youngest, Tori, has provided Helen with a rare perspective of the world. Tori has down syndrome and has brought Helen such joy in its simplest form. Although days are full there is a quieting of the soul and an alignment to being fully present and experiencing gratitude through her daughter's eyes.

Helen's audacious dreams include financing and working on ocean cleanup projects, developing a branch of her Arbonne business for special needs adults, and running a foster program for senior dogs. Research is underway now to open a plant-based B&B in Nova Scotia when the time is right for her family.

(416) 795-6496
Email: helenjsnell@gmail.com
Facebook: https://www.facebook.com/helensnellveganbeautynutrition/
Instagram: @helenharwoodsnell
Website: www.helenharwoodsnell.com

Love Transforms

By Anna van Dyk

When the unexpected happens, it can change your life forever. That's what an autism diagnosis did for my family and for me. Although I am extremely grateful for my son, it doesn't mean that the journey has been easy for us, especially since we had never encountered the word "autism" before. I am honoured to be able to share some things I have learned along the way. To get a better understanding of my story, a little background is necessary.

I graduated with a Bachelor of Science in Nursing in 1995, and soon after, married the love of my life. Together we decided to run our farm business together and raise a family. We were blessed with five beautiful little girls within a nine-year time span; life was very busy and very full. I remember quite distinctly having my life planned out for me. Then, our firstborn son arrived. At almost 10 pounds, Jeron's birth was difficult but he arrived safely and with just a tiny bruise on his head. All seemed well at first. He nursed well, gained well, interacted with his family and loved to cuddle. Jeron's development was no different than his five sisters.

Things began to change slowly after I stopped breastfeeding him at 14 months, and he was started on store-bought milk. He began to regress into his own world. He stopped babbling, we lost eye contact with him, and he began to display some behaviours we never saw with our other kids. One concerning thing was that he seemed to be addicted to the milk. He cried constantly for a bottle and would have at least four bottles of milk during the night. He had previously been sleeping through the night, but that wasn't happening anymore. He would need to be in his swing for hours at night after he had his bottle and he began to rock his head back and forth in a very odd way. It was like he was on a high. By the time he was 18 months old, he wouldn't care if I was in the room or not and wasn't talking at all. My family doctor was reassuring and sent him to speech therapy. In the meantime, my husband started looking into things himself to figure out what was going on with our son. After a couple of speech therapy sessions, the speech-language pathologist strongly suggested that he go and get a more thorough assessment with a pediatrician. Finally, Jeron was diagnosed with autism spectrum disorder at the age of 21 months, something my husband suspected, but I denied.

I could write many chapters about what happened in the months and years after his diagnosis; all the treatments, therapies, successes, and failures. You name a treatment or therapy, and I bet we've tried it in our attempts to "heal" our son. I dove into the research, read many books, and attended conferences across the country, all for the sake of finding that elusive "cure". I want to share something else with you—it's almost a confession. I wasted too many years and too many tears on trying to "find" my son and "get him back". The truth is, he wasn't lost. He didn't need the fixing—I did. In solidarity, my intention is that these next recommendations may help parents and caregivers on a similar path, and make the journey a little easier.

Allow Yourself to Process

After Jeron's diagnosis, I grieved and it was a very lonely time. I went through all the stages of grief and cycled back and forth through them many, many times. I bargained with God, I was angry, sad, and depressed. I said, "God, if you cure my son, I will travel the world and glorify you and share my testimony of healing." I was really struggling to get a handle on what was going on with my life and why it wasn't going as I had originally planned. To top it all off, we were also going through some other losses in our lives, and it seemed like we were on an endless downward spiral. As I hit rock bottom, I figured out I couldn't rely on myself like I was so used to doing. I had to rely on something so much greater than myself, or any doctor, expert, or specialist. I realized that God wasn't just for Sundays, put down my research and science books, and dove into spiritual writings and words of others to figure out how God was working in our lives.

After Jeron's diagnosis, I had to grieve all the hopes and plans I had for my firstborn son. I had made up stories of what his life was going to look like, and I struggled to give these up. Grieving is a healthy part of the process, and understanding that although an autism diagnosis seems like a loss, it is also a gain to something bigger and more beautiful than you can realize. Re-framing this is no easy transition, but it's something that I know you will also need to decide. With trust and openness, I slowly realized that God had a very different plan for our lives; better than I could have ever imagined. Although my original prayer was "God, fix my child", I started to take comfort in the verse from Jeremiah, "For I know the plans I have for you... a future full of hope"—Jeremiah 29:11 - 29 NIV; KJV.

While Jeron was in intensive behaviour therapy, we never imagined he would ever be able to handle going to school. Thank God he did, although it took two years to get him there full-time. When Jeron was in the primary grade, I would pick him up at lunchtime so we could have some one on one time together before everyone else came home from school. On those afternoons we would often walk in the fields. One day we were walking in a new area of the field, where sheep were grazing in the distance. Jeron picked up a branch that resembled a tall walking stick and tapped it on a rock, seeming to imitate Moses in the bible video he had been watching. This really caught my attention because Jeron, like many others on the spectrum, did not have the ability to imitate at that age. Suddenly, a song that I had learned when I was at his age came into my mind:

> "Moses tended sheep, upon a mountain top, he hardly noticed when a burning bush said stop, 'Set my people free and take them to my land'. That couldn't be my God they said, He'd have another plan. Well, Surprise, surprise, God is a surprise, right before your eyes, he's baffling to the wise. Surprise, surprise, God is a surprise, open up your eyes and see." —*God is a Surprise*, Rev. Carey Landry, Bloom Where You Are Planted, Songs of Faith and Growth

This affirmed to me that God did indeed have another plan for my son and for me and through His grace I was able to see clearly who my son is and what gifts he has to offer the world.

Trust Your Instincts

Instincts play an important part in any parenting, but when it comes to parenting a child with special needs, they are critical. Often parents become powerless and fearful when it comes to making decisions for their child, preferring to rely on the "experts" to make the decisions. However, as parents, we have an innate knowing of what is best for our children. We need to be able to tap into this knowledge, for the sake of ourselves, our child, and the greater good. To facilitate this, try finding a quiet place and spending time alone in order to get "in tune" with yourself. One example I can think of was the inner pull I felt to take the Kids Coaching Connection Course and become a life coach for children. I had all sorts of logic why I shouldn't take it and tried to talk myself out of it, but I could not shake the feeling that I really had to do it. I am so incredibly thankful that I listened to that inner voice and took the course. It was exactly what I needed. In teaching me to become a coach, it helped me become a better parent and served as an intense time of personal improvement and self-learning.

In one part of the course, we were coached to discover our Divine Design—our own life purpose statement. I discovered that my Divine Design is based on social justice and inclusivity for youth and families, and an opportunity showed up immediately after I claimed it. Out of the blue, a grandfather with his teenage grandson on the autism spectrum literally appeared at the door to where we were taking the course and wondered what we were doing. The leader of the course skillfully explained that once you claim your life purpose, the universe brings opportunities to you in alignment with it. Only in acknowledging and trusting my instincts was I able to take part in this life changing experience.

Instincts often have greater power than any logic or expertise, so we must listen carefully to that inner voice when making decisions for ourselves and our children. Not only must we trust our own instincts, but we must respect and trust those of our children. Kids have their own knowing too, which can be hard for a parent to understand—especially when a child is a nonverbal autistic. Jeron loved electronics and especially loved going on the internet and looking up all sorts of things. On the outward level, it looked like we had a bit of a problem on our hands with too much screen time. One day when my husband told Jeron he needed to get off the computer he responded with, "I have important things to do and this is important to me". Flabbergasted at the full sentence our nonverbal child just said, we had no choice but to honor that wisdom of his.

Jeron also used music he found on the internet to communicate with us. The first songs he kept repeating to us on YouTube were "Lead Me" by Sanctus Real, and "Home" by Phillip Phillips. Through these lyrics, Jeron was able to communicate and create his vision to provide a place for kids and people like him. That's how Spectrum Acres was created, a farm where all neuro diversities and abilities are welcome, accepted and loved for who they are in a natural, sensory-friendly environment. It all began with these songs, and to this day Jeron still uses scripts and music along with his own words to communicate with us.

When his brain doesn't allow him to use his own words, we use a letterboard from Spell 2 Communicate to really figure out what he wants to say. This mode of communication has been quite a learning experience for us and a whole new way to learn about our amazing son and what his thoughts and feelings are. Only by following my young son's lead were we introduced to this mode of communication serendipitously at one of the fun family events we hosted at Spectrum Acres. In trusting our son's own knowing and instincts, it has continued to help him reach his God-given potential.

Manage Your Energy

Jeron taught us very early on to be aware of our own energy and what we give off into the environment. Energy affects our kids all the time. They are emotional barometers; absorbing and reflecting other people's energy. My husband and I could be having a discussion in another area of the house, and if Jeron perceived that it was intense he would start to complain, fuss, and whine. When he was a toddler he would seek us out with his hands covering his ears and vocalize his displeasure of our discussion, only calming down once we had stopped. Jeron's sensitivity taught me the importance of taking a big breath during challenging situations like a tantrum or meltdown, instead of reacting reflexively. It also taught me that self-care is a huge necessity in order to manage our energy as parents.

Like many mothers, I too often put myself last on the list of priorities. When I am feeling well-rested, fulfilled, and content, Jeron shows it in his behaviour and so does the rest of the family. By modeling how to manage my own energy, the rest of the family naturally follows that example. We must also manage the energy that surrounds us in the environment by choosing what we expose ourselves to. The reason we spent so much time outdoors walking the fields was that Jeron did better when he was out in nature; the natural environment has its own calming and healing effect.

Because of Jeron's sensitivity, we had to be very aware of where we took him and who came into our home. Jeron could not handle going to a mall or grocery store—anywhere where there were a lot of people for many years. My daughters could not have friends over for sleepovers because Jeron could not sleep with the different energy they brought into the house. We really had to adapt our life to accommodate his needs and try to keep him in a regulated state. Further, we made sure we monitored his exposure to wifi and dirty electricity.

To this day we have maintained a wifi-free zone at home and aim to keep it that way. Not too long ago, one of my daughters decided she wanted wifi and bought a converter, plugged it in and didn't tell us. Suddenly Jeron couldn't sleep through the night anymore, and started to show some behaviours we hadn't seen for a very long time. After she came clean that she had plugged a wifi converter in, we removed it and Jeron could then sleep through the night as he had been doing. Energy is a mysterious thing, but we can help our sensitive kids by managing both personal and environmental energy.

Dare to Be Open

When parenting a child that is nonverbal or unreliably verbal, observational skills and "detective work" become so important. The behaviours your child exhibits are cues to what may be going on on a physical, mental, or even spiritual level. When Jeron was first diagnosed I became skilled at figuring out what Jeron needed physically. For example, I knew when too much sugar crept into his diet. He would be up in the middle of the night giggling to himself in what is called a yeasty laugh. Taking out sugar and upping the probiotics would make that disappear. It is easy to chalk behaviours down to the autism diagnosis, but being open and aware of the different things that may be causing them will vastly help your child. There were behaviours that he displayed that couldn't be explained at a physical level and I had no choice but to look at the bigger picture.

Jeron seemed to have a connection with the unseen world and often would call out to St. Michael when he was scared. He also would look in the distance and point past me and say "angel", and seemed to know things ahead of time. When I was only a few weeks pregnant and didn't even know myself that I was carrying twins, he looked at me one morning when he woke up and said "Hurray for babies". Shocked, because we had not told anyone yet, I quickly replied, "Pardon?". This time he looked right in my eyes and with a mischievous grin and repeated "Hurray for babies", emphasizing the word babies. An ultrasound a few weeks later did indeed confirm that I was carrying two babies.

These events could not be explained by my prior ways of thinking, prompting me to dig deeper and seek coaching and mentoring from professionals who had experience with this. As a result, I became a Kids Coaching Connection Coach and an Awesomism Practitioner. Through these experiences, I learned so much about Jeron, past the diagnosis, ultimately changing my relationship with him. Awareness and willingness to look at your child in different ways facilitates a new understanding of your child, which then allows them to be all they are meant to be in this world. I am grateful for the coaching, mentoring and training I had from these amazing people and highly recommend other parents to seek guidance in understanding your child. By this new level of understanding your child can move forward to their true potential.

Choose Love

It is said that love is a child's first language and that doesn't change for children with special needs and abilities. Our children teach us about "agape"—true, selfless, sacrificial, and unconditional love; a generous love that places the good of others over oneself. Jeron wanted me to share this quote from Thomas Merton: "The beginning of love is the will to let those we love be perfectly themselves. The resolution not to twist them to fit our own image. If in loving them we do not love what they are, but only their potential likeness to ourselves, then we do not love them. We only love the reflection of ourselves we find in them" (Merton, 2010). I challenge you to embrace this love and let it transform you.

Having a child with autism is not easy by any means, and it is easy to get stuck in the negative. Just like love is a choice, every day is a choice to let positive or negative thinking rule your relationship and interactions with your child. Choosing to let love rule opens the opportunity for amazing things to happen. For example, my desire to serve the unique mental health needs of those on the spectrum and their families has led me to go back to school to obtain my Masters of Social Work. Only through embracing my love for my son and those on the spectrum has this opportunity presented itself.

Oftentimes this love serves as a wake-up call. Because of our experience with Jeron's reaction to dairy when he was first introduced to it, we had a choice to make as dairy farmers. Learning about the negative impacts of A1 beta casein in dairy products through all the studies we read, caused us to undergo a huge change in our business. We began changing the genetics of our herd nine years ago to make sure our milk that we produce contains only A2 beta casein, which is not associated with the harmful effects on sensitive individuals, such as those on the autism spectrum. Without Jeron, we would not have even known about this issue with dairy and moving forward we will continue to educate and advocate for consumer choice of A2 milk in Canada.

Love is transformative. Choosing love over fear or anger has allowed us to be the best versions of ourselves. Parenting from a place of love creates all sorts of possibilities and creates a limitless space for God to work in your life. Through this love of your child, you will find your common mission and life purpose and be all who you were called to be.

It has been over 10 years on this off-road journey, with many bumps on the way—all opportunities to learn. I've learned along the way that the more trusting I am, the easier the road becomes, which allows for many blessings to occur. Going forward I can still glorify God through this life with an autism diagnosis and it's challenges. None of the blessings on this journey would have occurred without Him in the center of my life and of course without the greatest teacher in the universe—my son.

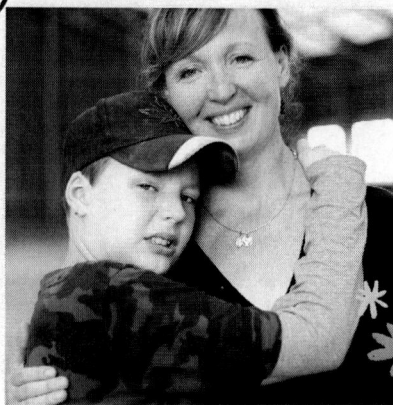

Anna van Dyk

Anna van Dyk is a mom to nine children, including a 12-year-old boy with autism spectrum disorder. Previously, Anna graduated with her Bachelor of Science degree in Nursing and was inducted into the International Honors Society of Nursing, then became a registered nurse. After the autism diagnosis Anna quickly began her journey into relearning and discovering what helps those with special needs actually helps the whole family. Through this, Anna became a Kids Coaching Connection Coach and Awesomism Practitioner. Combining her love for children, animals, and nature and through her son's vision, Anna cofounded Spectrum Acres. This led them both to coauthor the book *Awaken Your Inner Hero*, a collection of inspiring stories of Canada's heroic youth. When not advocating for and assisting those with autism and their families through coaching and events at Spectrum Acres, Anna is milking cows on the family run dairy farm with her husband. Since their son's diagnosis, the couple has revamped the way they farm and now are proud producers of A2 milk for people who are sensitive to A1 milk like their son. Now, Anna is also pursuing and advocating for the need of affordable A2 milk and infant formula in Canada.

Facebook: https://www.facebook.com/spectrumacres/
Instagram: spectrum.acres.perth.east
Email: annamvandyk@gmail.com

SECTION THREE:

A Special Needs Family "Healthy Life" Guide

This section of the book was the original idea for my book. I wanted to share all of the therapies, supplements, ideas we worked through over the years. I thought it could perhaps save someone the effort of having to dig deep online to find it all like I had to do, one by one.

So, to keep true to the original vision, in addition to all the amazing information shared by the co-authors of this book, I am going to keep this part here for you to use as you see fit. Take the parts that resonate with you and test them out. I am a firm believer that since everyone is unique, the solutions are also going to be unique.

Living Without Labels

In a world that is defining more and more physical and mental illnesses every year, it's my personal opinion that we (and I mean "we" as a medical/psychological professional "we") are tending to overly group and label our children. Why is this happening? Well, there are a few possible reasons that have crossed my mind:

1. We are labeling as mental illness what are really psychological states of being that were previously considered normal. Perhaps we've gotten better at detecting mental illness, and doing so earlier in the course of the illness. Therefore, if we are better at spotting it, we can treat it. For example, people who decades ago may have had undiagnosed attention deficit hyperactivity disorder, are now more likely to have their problems recognized and diagnosed.

2. Maybe there truly are more cases cropping up everywhere.

3. Or then, what was once considered psychologically healthy (or at least not unhealthy) is now considered to be mental

illness. Some of the behaviors, thoughts, and feelings that were within the "normal" range of human experience are now deemed to be in the pathological part. So, the actual definition of mental illness has broadened, creating a bigger umbrella with more people under it.

The normal trials and tribulations of life—the times of sadness, or worry, or anxiety, or grief, or difficulty sleeping, or drinking too much caffeine, or having caffeine withdrawal headaches—have now been pathologized. They've been made into mental illnesses.

Pharmaceutical companies search for an ever-wider market for their products. So it would make sense that when more people are diagnosed with a given disorder (perhaps because of less stringent criteria), or a new diagnosis is created, it widens the market for drugs. They push for "off-label" uses of their medications that in some way reduce a problem, and then they push for that "problem" to be redefined as a *problem* officially.

In our society of instant gratification, if a medication will help lessen uncomfortable thoughts or feelings or behaviors, we are more receptive to medication. Certain diagnoses—along with other criteria—make people eligible for government services or programs or supplementary educational services, or allow them to claim legal rights of nondiscrimination. People who feel they or their loved ones could benefit from those services may advocate for a widening in criteria that enables more people to be diagnosed and thus eligible for those services.

As our lives become more frantic and our workload becomes ever greater, having a diagnosis gives a name to the suffering we feel, and the hope that with a label can come relief. In challenging times, hope is essential. But, I'm not confident that labeling half of us with a mental disorder is the best way to give people realistic hope. So what's the big deal? So what if more people/children are being labeled and diagnosed these days?

I have a few reasons that I like to bring up while cautioning parents about labeling. It is so important to recognize that our children are so much more than diagnoses and conditions. In a society that is defining more and more physical and mental illnesses every year, we are tending to group and label our children. I do recognize that this labelling does come with it's benefits in our society. It allows us to receive help both financially and socially when we don't know how to help our children ourselves (behaviour issues, learning challenges, etc.). Without the label, the children tend to fall through the cracks of our education and medical systems.

However, I dream of a world without the labels, and encourage every parent who can avoid having the label attached to their child at a young age to do so. Often, parents report that their children suffered because they were not expected to excel due to their "label". Some children that I interviewed in the past reported "not trying" anymore because they didn't have to. They knew it wasn't expected of them.

This I can attest to personally with Johan. People around him tended to underestimate his abilities. Some people in the past almost seemed like they preferred him not to try new things, or activities that required extra support. It broke my heart when I saw that happen. There is no doubt that Johan wants to feel safe. But what I also grew to understand, was that when we did push him into new activities and challenges, he started to shine even more. He would amaze himself! And you could see him smiling, clapping, and laughing with complete joy at his accomplishments.

If we focus on the child and their abilities and work at nurturing what they are good at, we tend to see them bloom. When we support them and encourage them and even push them past their comfort zones, we can see them live to their fullest potential.

Energy Shifts

> *"Just like a single cell, the character of our lives is determined not by our genes but by our responses to the environmental signals that propel life."*—Bruce H. Lipton, The Biology of Belief: Unleashing the Power of Consciousness, Matter and Miracles

Our emotions are the language of our subconscious minds, influencing our cells in ways we're only just beginning to understand, and the placebo effect is a prime example of this. So, I feel it's important to share this information here for the sake of our special children. Why? Because after the diagnosis for my son, it felt very much like he was being placed in a very small box. So limiting.

And yet, he is so much more than his diagnosis. When I read Dr. Bruce Lipton's book, it gave me hope. Let me explain a bit about it.

The Biology of Belief explores how cells receive and process information. Implications of this research radically changes our understanding of life, showing that genes and DNA do not control our biology. Instead, DNA is controlled by signals from outside the cell, including the energetic messages emanating from our positive and negative thoughts.

Our thoughts. Wow! This was truly a life changing moment for me when I understood this concept. And not just in a "woo-woo" way (that's how some people refer to this type of topic when I have shared in the past). Dr. Bruce Lipton was going into the science of it all.

I mean, for decades, genetic determinism—that is, the idea that our genes are fixed, immutable, and outside of our conscious control—was the prevailing view of the scientific community, but now researchers have demonstrated that DNA is actually controlled by signals that come from *outside* of the cell. This is so important.

In other words, the cell's environment matters much more than we once thought. So, in theory, if you change the cell's environment you can change the cell behavior and genetic characteristics. Some of the most powerful external signals that influence the health of our cells are the energetic messages which emanate from our thoughts and feelings. Positive or negative (you have to really remember that it goes both ways), our thoughts have the ability to literally change our bodies and alter our physical health and well being. And this was great news for me to hear, because it meant that Johan was and is truly more than his diagnosis.

The Science of Epigenetics

Epigenetics is the study of cellular and physiological traits, or the external and environmental factors, that turn our genes on and off, and in turn, define how our cells actually read those genes. It works to see the true potential of the human mind, and the cells in our body.—Bruce Lipton (www.brucelipton.com)

Epigenetics is the science of hope in my world. When doctors, psychologists, and whomever else seemed to be counselling us at the time gave us dark and depressing outlooks on Johan's future, epigenetics gave me hope—we are more than our genes. Our external environment can actually turn our genes on and off. So, if there were some genes that were presenting themselves as "off" at birth for example, then I could introduce external changes to influence Johan's body's ability to turn them "on", and vice-versa.

Epigenetics is the field of study focused on how the environment influences genetic expression; it tells us that our nutrition, stress, and emotions can modify our genes. Now, what do we mean by environmental influences? It is everything that we do day-to-day. The food we eat or don't eat, the thoughts we have, both positive and negative,the air that we breathe, the way we move our body or don't move our body, and so forth.

Break that down into something even easier to understand: we have a BIG part in influencing our health and well-being, no matter what our genes might say. This meant, in theory, I could influence how well Johan developed and maintained his health and well-being by focusing on our lifestyle and making the necessary changes to support him as much as possible. And I am going to share some of the easiest ways I discovered to do this in the next sections.

Healthy Smells Good!

If I am able to make such an impact on Johan's life by making changes to his lifestyle, where does one begin? I mean lifestyle is everything. And everything is overwhelming.

The number one question I get from other concerned parents is always, "Where do I start?" Through the years, I have discovered how essential oils have the power to truly change your life! They are an easy first step to transform how you care for yourself and your family. They aren't just strange bottles that only certified aromatherapists know how to use—they have been around for ages.

Why did I make the changes in our home and lifestyle? I was tired of what the industry told me was safe. I was tired of government approvals of products that should never be in anyone's home. I was tired of wiping down my counters with bottles that say they are poisonous. I was tired of getting a headache when I walked by the cleaning aisles of local stores. And I was tired of worrying about everything in my home that could be potentially doing Johan harm.

I ended up ditching all sorts of harsh toxic chemical based products in my home and making it a safer place with plant-based alternatives. Johan had asthma. I say that he "had" it, because this is not something I have to worry about anymore in my own home—no guarantees when he is outside of our home, but at least I know it is safe here now. Every cleaning product, his personal care products, supplements, day-to-day needs, they are all taken care of now with essential oils and other plant-based products. And the difference is amazing.

I find children in general are drawn to essential oils. My youngest one has had them in his life since before he was born. And at only eight-years-old, he uses them daily for so many aspects of his day-to-day life, from school to sports to sleep, and so on. The important thing to remember is that everyone is unique. So take it slow. Allow your children to get introduced to the oils at their pace. To understand the full benefits of essential oils, you need to experience them. I could talk about them all day, but until you get to smell them and feel them on your body, you won't fully understand. So do yourself and your family a favour, research essential oils. I personally have only one company that I will use, because they produce the highest quality essential oils in the world. Check out our resource section for more information if you want to look into this some more.

I love this topic so much that I also wrote another book to help families get started called *Special Needs Essentials—The Go-To Handbook on Essential Oils.*

Fueling the Body and Mind

When the body has the right "fuel" it can soar! It tends to be such a key concept that is so challenging to follow through. I have found over the years that one of the common challenges with our special children is ensuring they get a healthy diet. Picky eaters, digestive issues, chewing problems, you name it. There are so many reasons why this can be a challenge.

For Johan, the biggest issue with food is that he does not chew. He also used to only drink out of a bottle. Unlike other children where the parents are running around making sure they don't put anything and everything in their mouth, Johan did not (and does not) like to have things near or in his mouth other than a reassuring finger that he often rests on his face. When he was very young, we went to nutritional counselling where they tried to get him to learn to chew by placing gummy bears in a mesh. He gagged. And personally, I wasn't too keen on the gummy bear incentive. Maybe I gave up too soon on this one, but he was determined not to practice chewing. So instead, I mashed everything up for him. For the most part, not a big deal. And really, it eliminates most "junk food". No pizzas and hotdogs, for example. Too much work to blend that up, and why bother? So, after understanding his preferences of having mashed foods which now are often more puréed than simply mashed, I began to focus on supplements. Food for everyone is less nutritious these days. Did you know that research has found statistically reliable declines for six nutrients—protein, calcium, potassium, iron and vitamins B2 and C in our food sources?

One key supplement that made the most significant impact in Johan's overall development, cognitive ability, and even his verbal ability was Auum Omega-3. It is a mammalian-source omega-3 supplement with additional vitamin D3 and vitamin A. We started taking it (I take everything Johan takes) when he was nine-years-old. I remember clearly the time that we got to test out the newest formula. After only about one week into the new supplement I asked Johan if he would like a snack. Normally, he would clap in happiness to acknowledge my question. Or, perhaps he would even nod yes, though less frequently and not consistently. But this day his face brightened up and he said in a clear voice, "Banana!". His favourite snack.

We have been taking Auum's Omega-3 supplement for over 12 years now. I know that his quality of sleep improved with it. His attention and focus increased a lot—so much so that his support worker and teacher at school commented on how alert Johan was suddenly. And he was responding to questions along with the rest of the class (not verbally, but with actions such as raising his hand to answer questions). I knew it was because of this supplement. Does he speak now? No. But he does verbalize a lot more than ever. We get many more words that we can understand.

And the biggest change? He wasn't getting sick as often anymore. And when he did, it wasn't a month or two off from school. He would get over things so much faster. Even faster than other children in his class. I am so thankful for this supplement. We call it our brain-food.

The Master Regulator

The brain is the "Master Regulator". What does that mean? Well, basically, if our body is a car, the brain is the driver. So taking care of our brain is so important. When I learned that Johan had issues with his brain, it took me down a very educational road. I never would have learned so much about the brain if it weren't for Johan. I would probably have taken it for granted like I did prior to his diagnosis.

The amazing thing that I learned is that the brain is more incredible than we even realize. If there is someone who says they understand all there is to understand about the brain, they are lying to you. We *still* know so little about it. The brain has a central role in the regulation of energy stability of the organism. It is the organ with the highest energetic demands, the most susceptible to energy deficits, and is responsible for coordinating behavioral and physiological responses.

And much like the hope that Dr. Bruce Lipton gave me through understanding epigenetics, Dr. Norm Doige gave me hope for Johan's brain through his book, *The Brain that Changes Itself.* In this book, he explains the term "neuroplasticity":

> *"The brain is not, as was thought, like a machine, or "hardwired" like a computer. Neuroplasticity not only gives hope to those with mental limitations, or what was thought to be incurable brain damage, but expands our understanding of the healthy brain and the resilience of human nature" (Doidge, 2008).*

So for Johan, I realized that even though there were issues with his corpus callosum and his myelin sheath, the brain is an amazing thing and there was potential for it to rewire itself in order to learn to work in different ways.

This then led me straight to Lee Gerdes, founder and CEO of BrainState Technologies™. I hosted a radio show for a few years and had the privilege of interviewing many wonderful guests (Dr. Bruce Lipton was one as well). When I received Lee Gerdes book, Limitless You, I originally thought it was a self-help book for the general population. When I discovered it was all about the brain, I could barely contain my excitement. It was like this was being given to me for a reason. Throughout the interview I could also barely contain my personal questions that I wanted to ask Lee for Johan's sake.

In the end I didn't hold back and we ended up talking about Johan and his brain. Lee was so fascinated by his condition that he invited us down to Arizona so that he could use his technology and check out Johan's brain and his brainwave imbalances. The trip to Arizona was a challenging one to say the least. I needed to fly down from Toronto with both my young children in tow. Johan was still incontinent. I was newly divorced and had no money. So, I borrowed from my mother in order to get there and find the cheapest hotel to stay in. I couldn't even afford a taxi to get around to buy food for our stay, so I walked everywhere in the scorching heat. I was exhausted and emotionally drained. But I needed to do this for my son. And I needed to keep it together for my daughter who was there to hopefully have a little fun despite all the massive changes that were going on in her life due to the divorce.

What we discovered during the Brainwave Optimization™ sessions was that Johan's brainwaves were really unbalanced! But what was truly exciting was how rapidly his brain waves were responding to the "brain training". Within just a couple of days, we saw immense improvements with some of the major imbalances that were discovered.

> *"By altering levels of brain energy through a feedback loop that allows the brain's own activity to be input into a computer and then fed back to it via auditory input, this advanced technology allows the brain to see itself—to recognize where it's out of balance and not functioning well. Once our amazing brain discovers how it has established neural patterns that may have been necessary for our survival in the past but that limit us in the present, it readjusts itself"* (Gerdes, 2011).

The week that we spent in Scottsdale, Arizona was just the start of my brain journey with Johan. I later went back and became a certified Brainwave Optimization™ technologist and opened up my own clinic here in Ontario, Canada. I needed to continue working with Johan's brain as much as possible. Things that I feel were directly impacted with this therapy were his incontinence (shortly after this trip he was able to understand a timed schedule for his toileting needs), and continued to support his cognitive abilities with speech and comprehension.

For those interested, I documented our journey in a video that you can find on my YouTube channel which I will include in my links.

It's a Gut Feeling

We have talked about the importance of food and nutrition. We have covered a little bit about our amazing brain. And now it's so important to talk a bit about the two together: with our gut health.

We hear a lot about eating healthy foods, proper nutrition, calories, and maybe we have even been told not to consume too much sugar. But what we don't always hear about and think about is the impact of what we eat on our gut microbiome. What is the gut microbiome? Your body is full of trillions of bacteria, viruses, and fungi. They are collectively known as the microbiome. While some bacteria are associated with disease, others are actually extremely important for your immune system, heart, weight, and many other aspects of health.

What does this have to do with the brain? The gut is physically connected to the brain through millions of nerves. Therefore, the gut microbiome may also affect brain health by helping control the messages that are sent to the brain through these nerves. These messages being sent by the gut may not control thoughts, but they do communicate with the brain in ways that may trigger mood changes. And it goes both ways. That is also why stress and emotional upset have a profound impact on gastrointestinal issues.

The gut is home to 70% of the immune cells in the body and 95% of the serotonin. Here are some potential symptoms to watch for in your child that may be a sign of distress along the gut-brain connection:

- Sleep problems
- Restlessness
- Irritability
- Headaches
- Tremors or shakiness
- Teeth grinding
- Procrastination
- Crying
- Nervousness

- Quick temper
- Depression
- Indecisiveness
- Poor concentration
- Trouble with memory
- Bloating
- Diarrhea
- Allergies

The gut microbiome is home to over 1,000 species of bacteria, and we need a healthy and diverse combination of both good and bad bugs in the gut. When that balance is out of alignment, symptoms can get worse. The exposure to toxic chemicals, antibiotics, drugs, and other substances have a direct effect on the gut flora. We know the importance now of protecting gut flora, and steps can be taken at any point in life to make beneficial changes.

Some key experts that I stumbled upon in my research for Johan's health are Dr. Amy Yasko (The Yasko Protocol), Dr. Keith Scott-Mumby (author of *Diet Wise: Let Your Body Choose the Food That's Right for You*), and Dr. Natasha Campbell-McBride (author of *Gut and Psychology Syndrome and the GAPS diet*). I highly recommend you check out their excellent resources and information to get a deeper understanding of the importance of diet and gut health and how it can impact our special children in particular.

The most profound experience Johan and I had with rebalancing our gut microbiomes (yes, me too! I do everything alongside Johan so that I can better understand what he is experiencing) was doing the GAPS diet. It is a highly restrictive diet that aims to heal the gut and reduce digestive symptoms rapidly. It requires you to cut out all foods Dr. Campbell-McBride thinks contribute to a leaky gut. This includes all grains, pasteurized dairy, starchy vegetables, and refined carbs.

I have never felt so depleted and weak in my entire life as I did during the first days of the GAPS diet! And I think Johan would agree. His eyes spoke volumes about his displeasure and disappointment each morning as his usual breakfast was replaced with GAPS-friendly options. He loves food so much, despite his chewing restrictions. And now, I eliminated so much off the menu!

Thankfully, the feeling was short-lived as our bodies did quickly adjust and new foods were slowly introduced back into our days. Did it help? I believe it did. We did three solid months of the GAPS introduction phase to heal our gut. It is recommended to go on much longer than that, however, I felt it was enough for us at this point. Since then we have continued on a very modified and healthy diet that avoids most of the foods that are considered less healthy for the gut. Johan's bowel movements have become much more consistent and healthy since then.

I do also caution you that this is not a diet to take on lightly. And if you have never done any type of detox or cleanse or modified diet, I probably wouldn't start with this one. There are many great resources out there to make it easier and safer. I purchased an entire "meal plan" guide that broke down the process into days. It provided exact recipes and timelines which were vital to my success with the program. You can check out the one I used by Cara from www.healthhomeandhappiness.com. Good luck if you decide to do this, and your gut will thank you.

To take your research into the importance of the gut biome even further, I highly recommend accessing the work of Dr. Zach Bush. Dr. Zach is one of the few triple board-certified physicians in the country, with expertise in internal medicine, endocrinology and metabolism, and hospice/palliative care. And one of his key topics of research that I feel strongly that everyone should know more about is glyphosate and the and many other dietary, chemical, and pharmaceutical toxins that disrupt our body's natural defense systems.

After studying his information for the past few years or so, it has solidified my understanding of the extreme importance of a healthy gut and how it influences the health of our whole body and mind. Since then, I have included a new supplement (not a probiotic) into our whole family's routine that was created by Dr. Zach called Restore.

The Immune System

Inflammation. I cannot complete this book without talking about inflammation and how it affects the immune system.

Here are some shocking statistics (sampled from the US):

- By 2011, the Centers of Disease Control (CDC) in the United States was reporting 54% of US children have some form of chronic disorder or disease by the age of seventeen, and these conditions occur in nearly every facet of the body—the hormone and immune systems, the respiratory and neurologic systems, and beyond. (https://www.academicpedsjnl.net/article/S1876-2859(10)00250-0/abstract)

- By 2016 the CDC reported 1 in every 14 children in the US have developmental disabilities, and 1 in 28 boys (1:28) have an autism spectrum disorder, and attention deficit disorder was found in one in ten (1:10) children. (U.S. DEPARTMENT OF HEALTH AND HUMAN SERVICES, 2017)

Why are so many diseases increasing at such a rapid rate? What's the relation? The connecting factor is chronic inflammation. And chronic inflammation is the root of all disease. To make matters worse these days we are spending more and more time indoors (usually in front of some sort of technology) and less and less time outdoors connecting with nature. And in a world full of harsh chemical disinfectants and cleaners, we are "protecting" our children from the dirt and bacteria that they need in order to be healthy!

According to Thom McDade, PhD, associate professor and director of the Laboratory for Human Biology Research at Northwestern University, our children's immune systems are actually strengthened by exposure to everyday germs so that it can learn, adapt, and regulate itself (Zamosky, 2014).

So let's bring the immune system back into this picture. Inflammation actually is the normal response of your body's immune system to injuries and harmful things that enter your body. Immune cells quickly react to the damaged area to fix the problem. So we really want to do everything we can to support the immune system so that it can function as intended and keep us healthy.

However, here are the top four things that reduce our immune system function:

1. Refined sugar—When you consume refined sugar there is an instant decrease in immune system function. Sugary junk foods gotta go. And,

even moreso, please do not drink it. Fruit juices, pops/sodas, energy drinks are best to be eliminated completely.

2. Lack of sleep—Everyone is unique, so the exact amount of sleep each individual needs to stay healthy varies. However, typically seven hours for adults and 10-12 hours for children. And please note that naps are not a replacement for quality sleep at night. They can be helpful, but the solid sleep during the night is key.

3. Processed food—The bottom line is that we are not designed to eat fake food. We need to change our thinking about the quality of fuel our body needs. We are the most incredible "machines" ever made and we need to treat our bodies properly. That means ditching the "fast food" and packaged pre-made foods where you have no control over what they are really made of. You need real food!

4. Stress—This is a tricky one because stress is something that typically most people experience. But what happens when we are stressed is the adrenal glands release cortisol and adrenaline and the immune system's ability to fight off antigens is reduced. That is why we are more susceptible to infections.

Now here are my top tips to helping to support the immune system:

1. Sunshine vitamin—Get outside and soak up the sun. Regular sun exposure is the most natural way to get enough vitamin D. To maintain healthy blood levels, aim to get 10–30 minutes of midday sunlight (between 10 a.m. and 2 p.m. to get the best of the UVB rays), several times per week *without* sunscreen (so important). People with darker skin may need a little more than this. Your exposure time should depend on how sensitive your skin is to sunlight.

    There are a few food sources that can provide some vitamin D3 such as egg yolks, wild salmon, and organ meats (do not reach for foods that claim they have added vitamin D3). And for those in areas that do not get a lot of sunshine throughout the year, a quality supplement such as Auum's Omega-3 with vitamin D3 (cholecalciferol) is key. This will help circulation, the sleep-and-wake cycle (meaning better sleep), and support lung health. It is a preventative measure for infections, cold and flu, hormone balance, metabolism, blood pressure, bone density, and overall immune function.

It is important to understand that our bodies contain cell receptors for vitamin D3 in virtually every system of the body. That means it is necessary for virtually all body functions. It influences the expression of over 200 health-supporting genes in our body and it lowers inflammatory reactions.

2. Sleep—During sleep, your immune system releases proteins called cytokines, some of which help promote sleep. Certain cytokines need to increase when you have an infection or inflammation, or when you're under stress (Olson, 2018).

There are many essential oils that can help support a relaxed environment and bedtime routine: Lavender, Tranquil, Valor, Peace & Calming, and Cedarwood are some of my favourites. Ensure there are no electronic devices in the bedroom (TVs, smartphones, iPads) and ensure the room does not have any light. Also, infrared mats that help to deliver negative ions to the cells and combined with amethyst quartz's conductivity has been shown to help with sleep issues.

3. Being active—When you move your body it helps to reduce stress, pump the lymphatic system, provides digestive support, and stimulates brain activity. Physical activity may help flush bacteria out of the lungs and airways.

Exercise causes change in antibodies and white blood cells which are the body's immune system cells that fight disease. So keeping our special children as active as possible is so essential for their immune systems. Walking is an easy way to boost your immune system if you can get your special child to walk for 30 minutes per day at least five days per week.

4. Fresh food—Fresh vegetables and fruits provide high antioxidants, packed with vitamins, and are beneficial in a myriad of ways. Antioxidants found in foods protect your cells from the effects of free radicals and can help reduce an overabundance of inflammation in your

body.

Fermented foods are a good way to increase the healthy gut bacteria which supports the immune system. A really simply one to make at home is wild fermented red cabbage. Wild fermentation is the ancient approach involving saltwater or brine exposed to the air. This results in thousands of species of bacteria, fungi, and viruses all intermingling into the fluid. They all work together to metabolize the cabbage or the miso, or whatever is being fermented.

There is actually a vibrational difference between processed food and homemade meals. The love and care that you put into making meals with real food increases the frequency of that food. High vibes are good for your health!

Incontinence

I would like to briefly cover the topic of incontinence here because it was (and still is in many ways) such a long-lasting challenge for us. I truly hope that some of this information might provide some guidance that might ease the journey for others with this situation (which for some reason has caused me the most daily frustration and stress over the years—not to mention the endless loads of laundry that it creates), and hopefully shorten the path to a working solution for your family.

I can still remember the dread I would feel waking up in the morning and walking down the hall to Johan's room, already being able to smell the strong stench of urine wafting up from under his door. At one point in our journey, this was part of my daily routine. This wasn't just an overnight incontinence that we were dealing with either. It could happen at any point of the day. It made school a stress. It made visiting people a stress. It made travelling anywhere (even short trips) a stress. Having spare clothes on-hand was a must. And doing laundry several times a day, everyday was the norm.

I remember feeling so frustrated, embarrassed, and guilty all at the same time. Reaching out to our doctor did not provide any answers. So once again, I was left to figure this out on my own. As the years kept passing and I was still buying diapers for my twelve-year-old boy, I started experimenting with many different methods to help with this situation. What I have really learned is that there is a fine balance that needs to be maintained with my emotions about this challenge. When I am super stressed about it, it also stresses Johan out. And when he gets stressed out about it, he starts to avoid drinking water because he knows that it makes him need to urinate. And he also holds it in longer, so the timing schedule gets messed up. So being prepared, being patient, being consistent with all the solutions that help support him has been the winning combination for us so far. And then on the days something doesn't quite work out, being understanding, towards both of us because accidents happen sometimes.

Essential Oils

We use therapeutic grade essential oils everyday in our home. Cypress, Geranium, and Juniper essential oils all have an affinity for supporting the urinary system and have been used for incontinence. Choose one essential oil, dilute with a carrier oil, and apply a few drops to the lower abdomen once or twice daily.

Another great oil protocol to consider is using a blend that includes Spearmint, Sage, Geranium, Myrtle, Nutmeg, and German Chamomile (over kidneys), and Cypress essential oil (over bladder) topically every evening to try to help balance out everything and support urinary health.

Copaiba is a powerful essential oil from South America that has traditionally been used to aid digestion and support the body's natural response to injury or irritation. Copaiba contains the highest amounts of beta caryophyllene (55%) of any known essential oil. To me, this is the best oil for inflammation which can be associated with incontinence.

Brainwave Optimization™

During my training with Brainwave Optimization™ I learned that possible causes of urge incontinence include dysfunction of the prefrontal cortex or limbic system, suggested by weak responses and/or deactivation, as well as abnormal afferent signals. So I focused on those areas of Johan's brain during his sessions as brain training sessions targeting those areas may help. To find out more about these types of sessions, you can learn more about the ever-evolving technology at www.cerest.com/legacy/.

Omega-3

Omega-3 fatty acids suppress inflammation in the urinary tract, which can help manage urinary incontinence and overactive bladder. Omega-3 fatty acids are required in every cell, as they play a key role in many essential processes. These range from the development and structural maintenance of nerve cells in your brain, eyes, and body periphery, to the anti-inflammatory effects they have in other cells of the body. We only use Auum Omega-3 supplements (mammalian source) because they are structurally unique to other omega-3 products (such as those derived from fish, algae, etc.) allowing it to be absorbed under the tongue (sublingually). This permits Auum Omega-3s to quickly enter the bloodstream, without first having to pass through the digestive tract.

However, in addition, Auum Omega-3's triglyceride form provides the ideal structure for absorption in the digestive tract, to allow for maximal digestion and absorption. Auum oil contains DPA, an omega-3 fatty acid not present in fish oils or other shelf supplements. This particular oil provides a full complement of omega-3 fatty acids, unlike any other.

Timed Toileting

A scheduled toileting plan is a strategy in which an individual is regularly transferred to a toilet, based on their individual habits. This seems like an overly simple solution at first glance. But it takes a lot of patience and consistency to get it to work. The great thing is that it does work for the most part.

Yes, there will still be times when "accidents" happen. And for us, certain situations or locations mean that Johan is not comfortable (too much noise for example) and it doesn't work. However, I found with the methods described above combined with timed toileting, my life has become a lot less stressful day-to-day. Going out into new situations, even at 21-years-old, is more challenging for us and I admit that I still get stressed with it. However, we have even managed to travel to destinations like Cancún, Mexico and Curaçao (which is even farther) from the Toronto Airport. These range from 4 to 6 hours of flight time plus all the extra time spent at the airports before and after the flight. Back-up clothing and adult-sized diapers are still always a must to have on hand for this type of travel since he will not use the airplane toilets at all.

Looking to the Future

This is probably the hardest section of this book to write because I feel I don't have all the answers that I need yet, let alone have the ability to share any advice with others. We are often reminded to live in the present moment and understand what a gift each day is with our children. Yet at the same time, as our children become adults, we start to realize the urgent need to plan for the unknown future. The future: what will it hold? There is no way that I or anyone can truly know. But there is one key question that I am certain every parent who has a child with special needs has asked themselves, "What will happen to my special son/daughter when I die?"

I have done such a thorough job up to this point in my son's life with his health and well-being, his education, his physical support, and therapies. As I continue into the routine that we have established for his day-to-day life, it becomes more evident that now is the time that I have to really start focusing on developing the connections and resources he will need in his life when I am not here to support him.

One of the main reasons that this is so important to me is that I want to ensure that it is my plan/solution for my son's life that is implemented and maintained, and not a government plan. My vision needs to be clear and concise. And my vision needs to be written down (in a will, preferably).

And this means addressing things such as establishing meaningful friendships for Johan. This to me is daunting because as many of us know, friendships are often not easy to come by for our special children. The relationships he has had outside of his immediate family have come from the schools he has attended. And primarily, he has made wonderful connections with his support workers. That is not to say that he did not interact with the other children in his classes. But the reality is, the friendships were temporary and based solely on the fact that they were in the same class. Johan has just recently graduated from high school, which means those connections are now complete as well.

In the past, we have been fortunate enough to have a weekend respite program that allowed us to have Johan stay over for two nights during the weekend a few times a year. Despite this being such a blessing, I can remember how nervous I was to leave Johan in someone else's care. However, those nervous feelings disappeared after that first weekend when I saw how happy Johan was there and how reluctant he was to leave. They paid so much attention to him. He had interaction with other children each weekend and the support staff. He got to do all the things he loved to do and more. And they fed him big meals! It got to the point where we would start pulling up the long driveway to the building where the respite was located and he would start to clap with joy. He knew he was in for a fun weekend. The staff loved him so much that he often got invited to stay for extra weekends whenever there was space available.

Since then, we haven't had the same luck in finding a place that was not only affordable (the weekend respite was a government funded program), but also that we felt truly comfortable with the quality of care they were able to provide. And quite frankly, we haven't found any place that was close to us now that we have moved to a new region. So our options for care outside of our home are extremely limited as we do not have any family members who can assist us either.

It is with full awareness that we start on this newest phase of Johan's life understanding the importance of establishing new friendships and connections for him. Potentially connections that will be able to outlast my own life. And I don't know how that will happen. And that concerns me. It also means that I need to start thinking of his ideal home as an adult. Right now I can't imagine him being anywhere but with me. However, down the road that may not be possible. What will that look like? What would make me feel comfortable and secure? What will be a good place for him to socialize and thrive? Will we have enough money to ensure he is in a good place? Are there some custom solutions that we can create for him such as cohabitating with other adults who have disabilities?

As I said, I do not have the answers for all of this yet. And many of the co-authors of this book aren't at the stage of even thinking about this phase of their child's life. I was so busy all these years focusing on the present moment, on the now, on his immediate needs, that I didn't take the time I now feel I should have to think about the future. Especially friendships and connections beyond the family.

So if this part of the book serves you in one way, I hope it simply makes you think every now and then about the steps further ahead. Not in dismay, but in a strategic way. That way, when your child is suddenly an adult, like my Johan, you are ready for what comes next in a positive and empowered way.

Personally, I find that when I do more research for Johan, it leads me to more hope. Right now, medically, Johan has some big hurdles to overcome. I feel strongly in my heart that we are on the verge of some massive shifts in our world, on so many levels, including medical advancements. I am also very hopeful that we will be coming together as a community more and more to support our children. When we work together and share together, we are strong together.

Closing Thoughts—The Power of Gratitude

As I look back on our story and read through all the others, one thing rings so true to me—I am so grateful. Grateful for having this crazy journey of ups and downs, of tears and joy, of frustration and success. It has all made me who I am today. I am so much stronger, wiser, and happier. Grateful for all the people that have come and gone along the way that helped and guided us. Grateful for the unsolicited advice from family, friends, and even strangers, because it shows that they noticed us and they care and they want to help in some way. Yes, there are still moments that I have all the emotions of our continuing challenges. However, they do not outweigh the good.

I am also so aware of the gratitude others feel for how Johan has touched their lives, even if it was only for brief moments in time. So many people have reached out over the years to tell me how much they love Johan and how much joy he has brought to their lives. For some, he was the reason they loved going to work each day. For others, he was the smile that brightened the room. And for others, he was the unconditional hug, or tickle, or laugh that reminded them that life is meant to be lived in joy. It makes my heart burst with pride and even more gratitude knowing how much he is able to share his gentle soul with the world in his simple ways.

I know that this is not the life that I envisioned for myself, and there may be times when I am saddened or stressed by some immediate challenge in front of us, however, I have also come to the point of my life where I am so grateful for all my children and all that they keep teaching me everyday. These days, one of the biggest challenges is finding ways to escape Johan's powerful bear hugs! He may be skinny, but he is so much stronger than he looks (inside and out). This challenge is one that I love and I understand how lucky I am to have this challenge each day.

So, if I could leave you with this thought to help you as you continue on your path—cultivate gratitude. It can be the saving grace for you and your special family. Write down all the things that are good in your life. Use words that uplift and empower you and your children. Surround yourself with people who bring you joy and words of encouragement and support. Share your successes with others to help others on their journey. Celebrate your child's wonderful uniqueness however you can.

"Gratitude is the heart's memory" —French proverb

Remember those in our lives who were there for us along the way. Remember all the wonderful moments that make your unique journey with your child truly special simply as they are, with all the ups and downs and loop-de-loops. This is the power of gratitude.

Recommended Resources

Over the years we have had very specific issues to work on and have come up with a variety of helpful resources, tools, and information that may be beneficial for your special child. Please note, we will have a much more up-to-date resource page with active links for your ease of use. You can access this list at www.fortheloveofourchildren.com

Reading List

Autism: A New Perspective, Inside the Heart and Mind of a Non-Verbal Man
– Andrea Libutti, MD and João Carlos

Awakened by Autism, Embracing Autism, Self, and Hope for a New World
– Andrea Libutti, MD

Biology of Belief, Unleashing the Power of Consciousness, Matter, and Miracles
– Bruce H. Lipton, PhD

The Crazy Makers, How the Food Industry Is Destroying Our Brains and Harming Our Children
– Carol Simontacchi

Diet Wise, Let Your Body Choose the Food That's Right For You
– Prof. Keith Scott-Mumby, MB ChB, MD, PhD

Essential Oils Integrative Medical Guide, Building Immunity, Increasing Longevity, and Enhancing Mental Performance with Therapeutic-Grade Essential Oils
– D. Gary Young, ND

The Infinite Possibilities of a Balanced Brain – Limitless You
– Lee Gerdes

Safe and Secure, Six Steps to Creating a Good Life for People with Disabilities.
– Al Etmanski, with Jack Collins and Vickie Cammack, RDSP contribution by Jack Styan

Special Needs Essential, The Go-To Handbook on Essential Oils
– Rose-Anne Partridge

Products

Juice Plus

Fruit & vegetable concentrate (in capsules, chewables):
https://sb23470.canada.juiceplus.com

Young Living Essential Oils

We have several co-authors that are Young Living Independent Distributors. Please reach out to the individual you would like to assist you in learning more about these powerful plant-based products and supplements.

Valerie Coates Distributor ID #14222809   (Co-Author Page 69)
Michelle LeRoy Distributor ID #1084801 (Page 8)
Isabel Neves Distributor ID #15487249 (Co-Author Page 104)
Rose-Anne Partridge Distributor ID #1318871 (Visionary of the book)
Laurie Sehl ID#17450230 (Co-Author Page 111)

Arbonne

For quality supplements, protein, probiotics, daily vitamins and more that are vegan, have no allergens, and no toxic ingredients, our co-author, Helen Snell, is about to assist you with Arbonne. Please visit her bio page for direct links to her Facebook page.

Services

Autism Ontario: advocates and a great resource for support, activities, outings and special events geared towards individuals in the autism community and their families.
https://www.autismontario.com/

Brainwave Optimization
www.cereset.com/legacy/

Kids Coaching Connection
www.kidscoachingconnection.com
Email: susan@magnificentcreations.com

(416) 708-6232

It has been proven that kids, youth and adults who have a positive sense of self, self-esteem and positive values have greater motivation to succeed, can deal with challenging life situations more effectively and will Manifest their Magnificence in the World. With the personal coaching services from Susan, we can reach the vast resources and powers lie within you.

Please contact Susan Howson for more information:

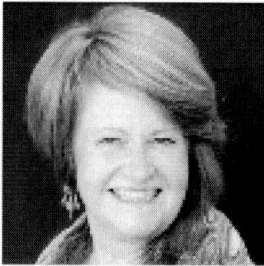

Susan is a leading edge Certified Life Coach, International Best Selling Author (Awaken Your Inner Hero and Dreaming Big; Being Bold), University Instructor, Metaphysical Minister, Speaker, Trainer, Social Entrepreneur, Tao Calligraphy practitioner and possibility thinker who inspires others personally and professionally. She connects people to their heart and soul, helping them Manifest their Magnificence through her products, coaching and training. She empowers kids, youth and adults to create a better world for themselves and others. Both her "Manifest Your Magnificence © " affirmation cards and fully approved International Coach Federation Kids Coaching Connection © program have won awards for their transformational impact.

Dr. Amy Yasko and the Yasko Protocol
www.dramyyasko.com

International Association for Spelling as Communication
Facebook: https://www.facebook.com/IASCspells/
Website: https://i-asc.org/

Our co-author, Anna van Dyk, is a certified S2C practitioner and anyone can find a practitioner close to them on the website.

Our co-author, Susan Baker's chapter is a great read to understand this practice for your child.

Jess Sherman
Nutrition strategies for autism, ADHD and anxious, agitated children
www.JessSherman.com

Julie Matthews
Science-based diet and nutrition strategies
www.NourishingHope.com

Ontario Autism Coalition: an integral group that unites the autism community and focuses on advocating for the rights of individuals in the spectrum.
https://ontarioautismcoalition.com/

Region-specific Resources and Programs

Precious Minds
Durham Region, Ontario life skills.
www.preciousminds.com
(905) 982-0882

Endless Abilities Inc.
Mississauga, Ontario therapy centre with an amazing team of behavioural therapists.
https://www.endlessabilities.ca/

Michelle Diaz-Jones: B.A. Linguistics, CDA Diploma, Reg. CDAAC
Speech-Language Assistant
https://sites.google.com/site/kidscommca/our-team

About the Author and Visionary of the Book

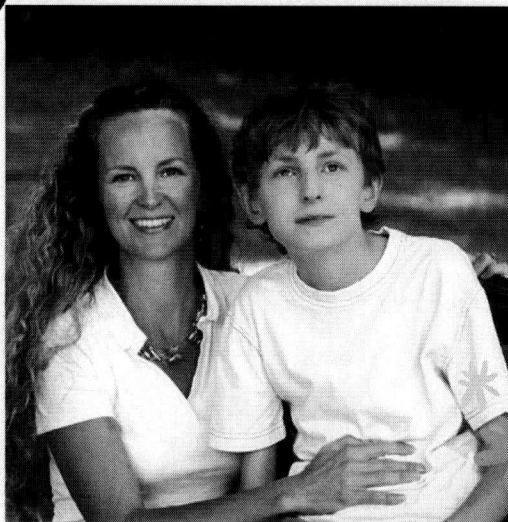

Rose-Anne Partridge is a published best-selling author, former radio show host and iTV personality. One of her most recent works includes co-authoring *The Power of Women United*. As a graduate of the University of Toronto, and after her son was born with a rare genetic condition, she went on to become an advocate and wellness coach for special needs and eventually founded Real Life Changes and Families for HOPE Network and Oily Masters. Rose-Anne continued studying brain nutrition and obtained her Brainwave Optimization certificate. She currently sits as a director of the Balanced Heart Mission (a community helping families with children who have autism) and has created a guide on how to use Young Living essential oils and related products to help our special children live to their fullest potential called, *Special Needs Essentials — The Go-To Handbook on Essential Oils*. Rose-Anne lives with her family in Ontario, Canada. You will often find her in cottage country enjoying the Canadian way of life.

Websites:
www.RealLifeChanges.com
www.SpecialNeedsEssentials.ca
www.FortheLoveOfOurChildren.com
www.EnergyLinkHealing.com
www.TheRightOmega3.com

Social Media:
Facebook: /OilyMasters, and /RealLifeChanges
Instagram: /reallifechangeswithroseanne and /oilymasters
YouTube: /reallifechanges

Email: roseanne@reallifechanges.com

References

Bethell, C. D., Kogan, M. D., Strickland, B. B., Schor, E. L., Robertson, J., & Newacheck, P.

W. (2011, May 01). A National and State Profile of Leading Health Problems and Health Care Quality for US Children: Key Insurance Disparities and Across-State Variations. Retrieved 2020, from https://www.academicpedsjnl.net/article/S1876-2859(10)00250-0/abstract

Doidge, N. (2008). *The Brain That Changes Itself: Stories of Personal Triumph from the*

Frontiers of Brain Science. Penguin Books.

Olson, E. J. (2018, November 28). Can lack of sleep make you sick? Retrieved October 07,

2020, from https://www.mayoclinic.org/diseases-conditions/insomnia/expert-answers/lack-of-sleep/faq-20057757

Gerdes, L. (2009). *Limitless You: The Infinite Possibilities of a Balanced Brain.*

Namaste Publishing.

Lipton, B. H. (2011). *The Biology of Belief: Unleashing The Power Of Consciousness, Matter*

& Miracles. Hay House.

Merton, T. (2010). *The Way of Chung Tzu* (2nd ed.). New Directions.

Zablotsky, B., Black, L. I., & Blumberg, S. J. (2017, November). Estimated Prevalence of

Children With Diagnosed Developmental Disabilities in the United States,

2014–2016. Retrieved 2020, from

https://www.cdc.gov/nchs/data/databriefs/db291.pdf

Zamosky, L. (2014, September 17). Are We Too Clean? Letting Kids Get Dirty and Germy.

Retrieved October 07, 2020, from

https://www.webmd.com/parenting/features/kids-and-dirt-germs